Better Body Workouts for Women

Dean Hodgkin

Caroline Pearce

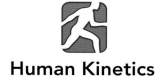

Human Kinetics

Library of Congress Cataloging-in-Publication Data

Hodgkin, Dean.
  Better body workouts for women / Dean Hodgkin and Caroline Pearce.
    pages cm
1. Exercise for women. 2. Physical fitness for women. I. Pearce, Caroline. II. Title.
  GV482.H58 2014
  613.7'045--dc23
                              2013013817

ISBN-10: 1-4504-3276-X (print)
ISBN-13: 978-1-4504-3276-4 (print)

The web addresses cited in this text were current as of July 2013, unless otherwise noted.

Developmental Editor: Laura Pulliam; Assistant Editor: Elizabeth Evans; Copyeditor: Joy Wotherspoon; Permissions Manager: Martha Gullo; Graphic Designer: Fred Starbird; Cover Designer: Keith Blomberg; Cover Model: Caroline Pearce; Photographer (cover and interior): Helen Roscoe; Photographer Assistant: David Rutter; Interior models: Caroline Pearce, Jenny Pacey, and Zoe Williams; Visual Production Assistant: Joyce Brumfield; Photo Production Manager: Jason Allen; Art Manager: Kelly Hendren; Associate Art Manager: Alan L. Wilborn; Illustrations: © Human Kinetics; Printer: Versa Press

We thank Premier Training International Ltd. (London Academy) in London, England, for assistance in providing the location for the photo shoot for this book.

Human Kinetics books are available at special discounts for bulk purchase. Special editions or book excerpts can also be created to specification. For details, contact the Special Sales Manager at Human Kinetics.

Printed in the United States of America   10 9 8 7 6 5 4 3 2 1

The paper in this book is certified under a sustainable forestry program.

Human Kinetics
Website: www.HumanKinetics.com

United States: Human Kinetics
P.O. Box 5076, Champaign, IL 61825-5076
800-747-4457
e-mail: humank@hkusa.com

Canada: Human Kinetics
475 Devonshire Road Unit 100
Windsor, ON N8Y 2L5
800-465-7301 (in Canada only)
e-mail: info@hkcanada.com

Europe: Human Kinetics
107 Bradford Road, Stanningley
Leeds LS28 6AT, United Kingdom
+44 (0) 113 255 5665
e-mail: hk@hkeurope.com

Australia: Human Kinetics
57A Price Avenue
Lower Mitcham, South Australia 5062
08 8372 0999
e-mail: info@hkaustralia.com

New Zealand: Human Kinetics
P.O. Box 80
Torrens Park, South Australia 5062
0800 222 062
e-mail: info@hknewzealand.com

E5742

I would like to thank and dedicate this work to my mother, who provides a source of constant inspiration and also has enduring faith in me, and my daughter, Imogen, who has helped me to realise that it's important to reciprocate a child's efforts in life to make parents proud.

—*Dean Hodgkin*

This book is dedicated to my parents, Chris and Jon Pearce. I love you so very much and thank you for your constant support and belief in me.

—*Caroline Pearce*

CONTENTS

Foreword   vii

Acknowledgments   ix

Introduction   xi

Chapter 1 **Training Essentials**   1

Chapter 2 **Fitness Assessments**   13

Chapter 3 **Nutrition Matters**   35

Chapter 4 **Warming Up
and Cooling Down**   51

Chapter 5 **All In Aerobics**   89

Chapter 6 **Go Anaerobic**   101

Chapter 7   **Going Strong**   **111**

Chapter 8   **Power Up**   **161**

Chapter 9   **Get Agile**   **191**

Chapter 10   **Personalise Your Programme**   **201**

Chapter 11   **Sample Workouts and Programmes**   **213**

Chapter 12   **Training Diary**   **235**

Appendix: Choosing Your Workout Clothing and Style   241

About the Authors   247

FOREWORD

A the editor of *Bodyfit*, one of the UK's leading women's fitness magazines, I'm exposed to all the latest trends in fitness and nutrition. Being bombarded with press releases about new products, foods, supplements and fitness protocols often makes it hard to interpret the sometimes-conflicting information presented. One day a certain diet or food is in vogue, and the next's to be avoided at all costs! So, when it comes to relaying the best information to my readers, I like to keep things simple, which is why *Better Body Workouts for Women* is great. It presents straightforward, step-by-step exercises suitable for both gym and home workouts, along with scientific know-how to back it all up.

In this addition to the Human Kinetics family, Dean Hodgkin (fitness expert who appears at events internationally and a former world martial arts champion) and Caroline Pearce (international athlete, sport scientist, presenter and former TV Gladiator) bring you all the tools you need to get into the best shape of your life. Dean has written extensively for *Bodyfit* since it was launched in 2010. He's covered training plans for all abilities and how to have your fittest year yet. Caroline, also part of the *Bodyfit* team of writers, currently showcases her top toning exercises on the Caroline's Core Moves page each month. With such a wealth of combined knowledge about sport, anatomy and fitness, the pair has created a guide to everything you need to know, and do, to make the body of your dreams become a reality. Beginners can get started with fat-burning and toning exercises, and more advanced exercisers, or even those thinking about becoming personal trainers, can find in-depth information about nutrition, anatomy and various fitness tests.

POWER OF THE MIND

It's not only physical exercises you'll find in this invaluable new guide. The authors address one of the most important subjects regarding weight loss and exercise, an area not often covered in health and fitness books but that is now coming to the forefront of mainstream wisdom: the mind–body connection. Dean and Caroline understand how your mental and emotional faculties affect your ability to achieve fitness goals. They offer guidance on tackling negative self-talk as well as what to do when you fall off the fitness wagon so you can get straight back on instead of beating yourself up—which we women are usually pretty good at! Getting into the right frame of mind, believing and feeling worthy of changing your shape, and staying focused and motivated are some of the biggest factors influencing your success. Lack of belief, feeling unworthy, or thoughts such as *I don't have time* all act as silent saboteurs to your progress. Deal with your mind first, then the physical side will have a better chance of transforming.

If you feel good about yourself, you're more likely to want to exercise. Of course, working out also boosts your endorphins and makes you feel better, putting you in a more positive frame of mind.

YOUR FIRST STEP TO FITNESS

So, there really is no reason not to leap into your exercise journey with Dean and Caroline helping you break down your goals into manageable short-term projects so that you're more likely to achieve those long-term targets, such as dropping half a stone or toning up in time for your wedding. It's the combination of all those little steps that adds up to huge physical change further down the line. So, the most important thing now is just to begin. Any journey starts with a single step, and you've taken that first step to maximising your fitness by buying this book. May you be well, happy and successful.

—*Katy Louise Evans*, editor, *Bodyfit* magazine
(www.bodyfitmagazine.co.uk, @bodyfmag)

ACKNOWLEDGMENTS

I am immensely grateful to Caroline Pearce, my co-author, for joining me on this journey and bringing an incredible depth of knowledge, far-reaching and admirable experience plus inspirational energy that, when combined, demand respect from all who are lucky enough to work with her. In addition, I wish to thank Karalynn Thomson for her efforts to get this project off the ground. Naturally, I wouldn't even be in this position without having been incredibly fortunate to have encountered many gifted and inspirational industry professionals along the course of my career, who imparted the knowledge and skills that enabled me to input to this book. Although too numerous to mention, I'm confident when reading this, they will know who they are.

—*Dean Hodgkin*

I would like to thank my partner David Godfrey, a trainer and NLP practitioner, for his advice and feedback throughout this project. Special thanks also to my former athletics coaches Ron Stern, Bruce Longden and Martin Green for providing such a solid foundation of training and education during my competitive years. I'd also like to thank Performance Health Systems and Power Plate International for providing so many opportunities for me to grow and gain experience around the world in the fitness and well-being industry as a master trainer, presenter and spokesperson. Thanks also to Karalynn Thompson for her early help with this book and to the Human Kinetics team, Laura Pulliam and Jason Muzinic, for their guidance and direction throughout. Lastly, it has been an absolute pleasure to work with and share this journey with my co-author Dean Hodgkin, whose experience, accolades and success in the industry are truly admirable and of great value to this book.

—*Caroline Pearce*

INTRODUCTION

Warning! This book contains advice for women who are serious about fitness. If you are not looking to dramatically change the shape of your body and your outlook, put this book back on the shelf and walk away!

Okay, so that's a bold statement to make, but it's only fair you know that this is not just another tome to sit alongside other titles in the fitness genre. Rather, this book is for the woman who is exercising regularly but who feels somewhat in a routine rut, or the one who has found that the law of diminishing returns has begun to apply, whereby she stops seeing results despite sticking rigorously to her routine. If this is you, then read on, as the solutions to all your problems are here.

Through a wide spectrum of scientifically proven techniques, this workout bible will take your training into a new dimension, providing the inspiration, education and motivation to lift you off your current plateau and accelerate your results. It presents information in a modular format so you can cherry-pick whatever you need, whenever you need it, and thus can easily adopt the various guidelines and assimilate them into your current lifestyle. Don't wait weeks for the next month's issue of your favourite workout magazine to hit the newsagent shelves in order to satiate your thirst for new direction. This is truly your one-stop shop for all that is fresh in fitness. Consult the book during workouts to ensure you religiously put into action the invaluable advice you'll gather here. Specifically designed with usability in mind, this book is conveniently sized to fit into your gym bag and is easy to clean in order to withstand the rigours of being dragged around the gym or exposed to the currency of hard work—sweat!

Research has shown one size doesn't fit all when it comes to exercise programmes. No two bodies are the same, so what works for one of your friends may not work for you. This is why the personal training industry sprang up and why good personal trainers often come with a considerable price tag attached. What you will find here, however, is an insight into the tricks of the trade. Think of this book as your own personal trainer toolkit, allowing you to design the ideal workout for you and you alone. Let's call it your perfect fit! As you work your way through the book, you will begin to learn more about yourself, particularly how your body works and, more importantly, how it responds to varying training demands. Clearly, understanding how improvements in your sports performance and silhouette are achieved will help you not only reach your goals sooner, but also maintain your higher ground.

In addition to introducing you to advanced training protocols to improve strength, muscular endurance and cardiorespiratory fitness (in the home, outdoor and gym environments), this book emphasises flexibility as an important component in both physical performance and general well-being. It also focuses on correct nutrition, recognising its importance for both deriving optimum benefit from your workouts and achieving the aesthetic goal of reduced body-fat levels that most of us aspire to. It even includes sample menu plans to help you to fuel like an athlete from day 1. Since a link clearly exists between exercise and reduced risk of a plethora of lifestyle diseases, this book also explores the pathology of such and the mechanics behind how regular exercise produces a positive influence.

Skill-related fitness components, such as agility and power, are often left in the pigeonhole of the elite sports performer. This book singles out these areas for special attention, as they help you vary your training programmes, thus maintaining your interest. Beyond purely putting the fun back into fitness, these sections will give you a greater understanding of holistic workouts and all-round fitness.

Summoning the motivation to make changes in your exercise and diet habits is central to attaining a meaningful degree of success. Here, you will explore this area, particularly the concept of setting goals. Learning how best to develop a framework for improvement carries substantial weight when you consider the old adage 'To fail to plan is to plan to fail!' A lot of people who stop exercising simply lack the right attitude. This section will help you to avoid becoming one of those drop-out statistics by teaching you the mental skills required to incorporate new workout concepts and lifestyle patterns. Once your head is in the appropriate place, you will be able to make best use of the text's fitness building blocks, so ensuring they will work for you in the longer term.

The authors bring a wealth of experience in many aspects of health and fitness, and both embody the principles they espouse. Dean Hodgkin has trained thousands of fitness instructors, managed health clubs and spas, worked as a consultant to leading sportswear brands, including Reebok and Nike, and appeared as a key presenter at fitness events in 36 countries. He received the International Fitness Showcase Lifetime Achievement award, was voted best international fitness presenter at the One Body One World awards in New York and won three world, plus two European golds in karate. Caroline Pearce is a former international heptathlete. She graduated from the renowned Loughborough University with a Master's degree in exercise physiology and nutrition and a first-class honours degree in P.E. and sports science. She was one of Sky TV's UK Gladiators and works as a television sports and fitness presenter, sports model and international master trainer for Performance Health Systems. In her master trainer role, she has guided everyone from celebrities to sports stars, trainers and government healthcare officials around the world. In addition, both authors are established writers, contributing to a wide range of publications from national newspapers to monthly magazines and trade journals.

Rest assured, then, that you'll find no padding here, no latest fads or dubious celebrity-endorsed practices. Every chapter contains factual information, workable plans, easy-to-understand tables and empowering statistics that you can immediately put into use. All this is backed up with tips so you can easily identify and then remember the most salient points. Never again will you struggle to differentiate between fact and fallacy, hit and myth. From here on, your workouts will put not only sweat on your brow, but also a smile on your face.

The journey to a new, fitter, slimmer you begins when you turn this page. So, what are you waiting for?

Training Essentials

We have assumed that those of you purchasing this valuable resource already possess a certain level of fitness knowledge, but we also recognise that you may have decided you wish to ramp up your efforts in order to achieve better results. Set aside a moment to take stock now. This chapter equips you with the basic understanding and skills for making a successful journey to a fitter you. It covers a myriad of related and unrelated components that can affect your workout routine. Although some of this may not be new, the content further develops understanding and provides motivation and a fresh approach to training.

THE MIND–BODY LINK

Let's begin by ensuring your mind is in the right place, as you'll no doubt be aware of the importance top athletes place on having a positive mental attitude. Self-talk, breathing exercises, meditation, guided imagery and visual rehearsal are all widely used tactics. One size doesn't fit all in this domain, however. You need to discover what will work for you to reach the next level of training, and you then have to commit to your set of cerebral ground rules.

Accountability

You are the one who must take responsibility for the success of your routine, specifically for avoiding excuses and circumnavigating obstacles in the forms of work pressures or family commitments. This also extends to your group exercise instructor and personal trainer if you have one, as you will be the one actually performing the exercises. You can gather all the support in the world around you, but the brutal truth is that only you can buy your success—and the currency is sweat.

Mantra

Henry Ford is quoted as saying, 'Whether you think you can or think you can't, you're right.' Start to tell yourself 'I can' or 'I will' every time the alarm goes off early, the last mile seems too hard, there are no repetitions left in your arms and you feel as though your tank is running on empty. You'll be amazed at what you can achieve by keeping this simple thought in your head. It might even pay dividends to write your own mission statement at the front of your diary so that you regularly remind yourself what you're doing, why you're doing it and where it will take you.

Consistency

Success is achieved by harbouring a constant desire for improvement. Whilst you will achieve your best results by varying your workouts to avoid the dreaded plateau effect, you will have to stick rigidly to your plan and to recognise that when external pressures throw you off course, you must strive to get back to your routine as soon as possible.

Work Ethic

You'll be familiar with the ubiquitous suggestion that anything worth having is worth working for. This saying applies 100 percent to improving your fitness. You will need to summon equal measures of willpower, persistence and discipline. Even then, you will have to accept delayed gratification. Rome wasn't built in a day, so they say. Rest assured, however, work hard and you will achieve incredible results.

Powerful Imagery

Take a moment to compile a picture montage of what fitness means to you, what you love about working out and how you think you'll feel when you achieve your goals. You don't need to be particularly artistic. Simply gather a variety of lifestyle magazines and cut and paste, in the old-fashioned way, to make a feature to be displayed in a prominent position in your home so you see it each day (finally, a use for those fridge magnets!). You could even split it into two halves, with positive, inspirational images on one side and negative pictures on the other to remind you of both what you're moving away from as well as moving towards.

WEIGHT-LOSS TIP Saying 'I don't eat junk food' rather than 'I can't eat junk food' is reported to make you eight times more likely to resist it. Saying 'I don't' gives you ownership of the idea, whereas 'I can't' suggests that something beyond your control is responsible for your actions.

PERSONALITY TYPES

The preceding information is all fairly sound, and we suspect you won't disagree with any of it. However, we all have different personalities, which will clearly affect the likelihood of maintaining the previous commitments. So let's take this head-on and tackle a few of the more common forms of the disease we like to refer to as 'excusitis'.

Pursuit of Perfection

This is the desire for everything to be just right before you embark on your new routine, from getting new kit and shoes to rearranging your diary in order to provide regular workout windows. You know things will never be perfect, so this is a way of dumping your accountability. After all, how can you be to blame if the weather was too bad for your run? The way around this barrier is to avoid an all-or-nothing approach; always have alternative plans. For example, if you really can't make it to the gym for your 30-minute workout one evening, try to slip in a 15-minute session before work and another one in your lunch break.

Fantasy Fitness

Dreaming about being in great shape is a common pastime for many women, but it is of little use without action to accompany it. It's vital to set short- and long-term goals using specific dates and concrete numbers, so the next section looks at this in detail. In addition, you need to have a clear plan of precisely what you're going to do every time you visit the gym, set off on a run or dive into the pool. A detailed plan allows you to measure yourself against your intended objectives for the session. This is crucial when reviewing your training diary (see chapter 12) in order to improve your efforts.

Don't Worry, Be Happy

Worrying about whether you can handle the step-up or really put in the time and effort, plus whether you honestly feel your goals are achievable are all negative thoughts that can lead to procrastination. The fact is that you are today where your thoughts and actions have led you, so you will be tomorrow where they lead you also. If you stumble upon a 'what if', think it through to its conclusion. For example, if you think you might not have it in you to complete a particular workout, think back to the last time you felt that way but still made it through. Also remember that even if you don't manage to accommodate the full routine, as long as you try your best, you'll be taking another step forwards on your journey.

The list of commitments introduced earlier makes it clear that you'll need to put a lot of effort into your new exercise routine if you want to attain the results you seek. This brings the issue of motivation into sharp focus. To stay motivated to succeed, adopt and adapt these top tips to keep your thoughts and actions true to the cause.

GOAL SETTING

Your next step is to identify your fitness and body-shape goal or goals. It's no use simply saying 'I want to be fitter or slimmer'; you need to be more specific. Likewise you have to be realistic. Unfortunately you won't lose 10 kilograms in the week before your wedding! The SMART model identifies the key components of setting a good goal:

- *Specific*—This is the what, why, how, where and when of your goal. For example your goal may be to shave 5 minutes from your 10-kilometer time (what) and to improve your national ranking and a place in the team (why) by following a training programme involving two endurance runs and two interval timed sessions per week (how) at your local track and park (where) every Monday, Wednesday, Friday and Sunday (when).

- *Measurable*—Choose a goal with measurable progress so you can see the changes occur. Take measures to check that you are on track and to know when you have achieved your goal. Measurable goals include achieving a racing time, lifting a particular weight, losing a set amount of weight, making the team or adhering to a specific training protocol or nutrition plan. Use the assessments in the next chapter to measure your progress across different variables related to your goal.

- *Attainable*—Be realistic when you set yourself a goal. Perhaps even involve a personal trainer, family member or friend to help you to do this. If you set a goal too far beyond your reach, you will start to feel overwhelmed and will lose belief that you can achieve it. This in itself can stop you from even giving it a try. However, your goal needs to stretch you slightly so you feel there is something to aspire to and to move you to make a real commitment. It is the feeling of success and accomplishment of the goal that will help you remain motivated. Remember, if you reach your goal sooner than you thought, you can set another, pushing the boundaries a little farther each time.

- *Relevant*—To maintain commitment to achieving your goal, the goal must be relevant to you. Adopting the same goal as a friend may not work for you, as your motivations and needs will likely differ. A relevant goal is one that has meaning to you and will enhance your life, belief and feeling of well-being. For one person, this may be to lose 5 kilograms of weight to look better and improve self-esteem, whereas for someone else, that same loss of 5 kilograms will aim to improve her strength-to-weight ratio and, thus, sporting performance.

- *Timely*—Your goal should be grounded within a time frame to gain a sense of urgency. This time frame needs to be specific. It's no use saying you would like to run a marathon someday. Instead, set a date and book your place in the race so that your unconscious mind moves into motion to guide your conscious mind to start planning and setting targeted steps towards your goal.

We'd like to also suggest an additional requirement to your goal setting: It should be revisable. We don't expect you to be spot-on accurate with the goal you set, especially if this process is new to you. You must be able to revise and adapt your goal in response to your measured progress towards it. Unforeseen circumstances such as illness or injury can alter the time frame of achieving your goal, whilst a realisation of its actual difficulty when set in motion, causing you to feel disheartened, may prompt you to reduce the difficulty level of your goal in the short term to make it more achievable. Life is ever evolving, and so should you be!

THREE REASONS TO SET FITNESS AND TRAINING GOALS

Despite the raft of research out there confirming that goal setting is vital if you wish to set yourself up for success, it is all too often overlooked. Just in case you're sitting on the fence, here are the key reasons why you should commit to this endeavour from the outset.

1. *Motivation*—When you're clear about what you're trying to achieve and you attain the mini targets set en route to your goal, then you are more likely to be motivated to continue.

2. *Focus*—Goals make you accountable to yourself and to others. Write your goal down and tell others about it to help you stay focused every step of the way. Without a goal, it is easy to stray off track and lose focus.

3. *Achievement*—Without a goal, how will you know if you have achieved anything? You may be able to make some general sweeping statements about improvement, but they will not be measurable or tangible. Reaching your goal is a clear sign of an achievement, a reward for your efforts. It leads to high self-efficacy, which enables you to believe in yourself and to keep improving.

Long-Term and Short-Term Goals

When you've set your ultimate goal, or your *long-term goal,* it's important to break it down into smaller targets known as *short-term goals.* These may be daily, weekly or even monthly targets that provide the stepping stones to your ultimate goal that will provide you with valuable feedback and motivation. Apply the SMART principles to both your short- and long-term goals. Here are two examples:

Example 1

- *Long-term goal:* to reduce your body fat by 10 percent and fit into a smaller dress in 6 months.
- *Short-term goals:* (a) to consume 1,600 calories per day for 6 days per week, with 1 day for allocated treats with a maximum intake of 2,000 calories, (b) to complete two cardiorespiratory workouts and two strength workouts, 1 hour in duration, every week and (c) to cycle to work every day and climb the stairs to the office rather than take the lift.

Example 2

- *Long-term goal:* to run a track 800-metre time of 2 minutes, 15 seconds at the club championships in September.
- *Short-term goals:* (a) to complete two over-distance time trial runs of 1,000 metres twice per month, (b) to race a 400-metre distance prior to the championships in under 60 seconds for test of speed endurance and (c) to improve running efficiency through completion of gait analysis testing once per month.

These short-term goals are specific and directly linked to the long-term goal. You may also set mid-term goals, which, as the name suggests, are set for the halfway mark en route to your main long-term goal.

Goal-Setting Template

The SMART model provides information on how to set goals and on the factors to take into account. To make sure you don't miss a step in the process, figure 1.1 shows a goal-setting template to complete or adapt to meet your needs. If we take the first of the previous examples, the table will look like the one shown in figure 1.1.

Figure 1.1 Goal-Setting Template

	Specific	Measurable	Attainable	Relevant	Timely	Achieved (list dates and tick off)
Long-term goal	Reduce body fat	Drop 10% on body-composition score	✓	✓	6 months	
Short-term goal 1	Consume fewer calories	Target 1,600 kcals	✓	✓	Daily	
Short-term goal 2	Increase workouts	2 strength and 2 cardio sessions	✓	✓	Weekly	
Short-term goal 3	Increase activity levels	Cycle to work	✓	✓	Daily	

BARRIERS TO FITNESS

Despite having the best planning and assessment techniques, sometimes life just gets in the way, and you allow it to prevent you from reaching your goals. We say 'you allow it' because you are always in control of your actions and accountable for what you do. Everyone faces barriers to fitness to some degree or another, but the key is to identify these barriers and overcome them. This process separates those who succeed from those who don't! But first you have to want to make a change or improvement—only then will you take our lead and follow our advice (but we're hoping as you're reading this book, you have already taken that first step and made the decision to reach the next level).

Here is a list of common barriers to training and to good nutrition, with our pick of the best ways to overcome them. Excuses will now be a thing of the past!

Lack of Time

With a full-time job, travel, work functions or overtime, family commitments, meetings and household chores to squeeze in, lack of time is the most commonly reported barrier to exercise. Solutions to your perceived lack of time might be as follows:

- *Get up earlier*—Simply reset your body clock to get up 30 minutes earlier three or four times a week to exercise. You will quickly adjust and find that the endorphin boost from early-morning exercise gives you more energy for the rest of the day.

- *Accumulate exercise*—If your goal is weight loss and improved health, simply adding more general activity to your day will help you achieve it even if you don't do a structured exercise plan. Walk the stairs and ditch the escalators and lift, leave your car behind or at least park it farther away from your destination and take a power walk during your lunch break.

- *Incorporate fitness on the weekend*—Why not use the weekend to catch up on your fitness and have fun at the same time? Swap your coffee mornings with friends for a power walk or cycle together. Rather than watch the kids swimming, get in the pool and join them. Try new activities with friends and family, such as climbing or kayaking.

- *Explore home workout solutions*—More home fitness solutions now exist than ever before, and they can be just as effective as a visit to the gym. These include workout DVDs, body-weight circuit sessions utilising the furniture (stairs for step-ups, sofa for triceps dips) and an all-in-one gym machine that can be stored away easily when not in use.

WEIGHT-LOSS TIP Research shows that sleep loss can lead to increased hunger levels the following day. If you're setting the alarm for an early workout, you will also need to hit the sack a little earlier to achieve a good number of total hours in bed.

Lack of Confidence

A surprising number of women avoid exercise because they are embarrassed about how they look and scared that others will judge them. If you're one of those women, rest assured that others are more concerned with themselves and their own workouts to be judging you—they probably have their own hang-ups, too. Solutions to lack of confidence might be as follows:

- *Avoid the crowds*—If you have the flexibility to choose your gym time, you will find fewer crowds mid-morning and mid-afternoon.

- *Begin at home*—If you want to make some progress before you hit the gym or park for your workout, begin with the home workout solutions mentioned previously. We've provided some great body-weight exercises you can try in later chapters.

- *Invest in some great workout clothing*—Buy a kit that fits right, breathes, removes sweat from the surface of your skin and covers the body parts you are most conscious about in order to feel the part and be more self-confident when working out.

- *Focus on the future*—Banish feelings of self-consciousness by reminding yourself of the cardiorespiratory and strength benefits you are achieving with every session. The more you exercise, the more confident you will feel.

Saboteurs

Sadly, others—friends, colleagues or even loved ones—act to sabotage your fitness or dietary efforts. Sometimes this is because of their own insecurities that you may leave them behind and start to look and feel better than they do. It can also be their own lack of understanding of your goals. Don't let others jeopardise your efforts. Solutions to these saboteurs might include the following:

- *Shout out your goals*—Tell everyone around you about your fitness and dietary goals and how important they are to you. Tell them how much their support means to you and even encourage them to join you on your journey.
- *Bring in back-up*—If colleagues or loved ones are stocking the cupboards to tempt you with sweet offerings, the last thing you want is to give in due to hunger! Make sure you have your own healthy snacks in hand and that you eat every 2 to 3 hours. We have some great snack solutions in chapter 3.
- *Surround yourself with positivity*—If others are bringing you down despite your attempts to inform them of your goals, then quite simply extract yourself from their company and surround yourself with those who do support and share in your desire to be fit and healthy.

Injury or Illness

Injury and illness are the most acceptable barriers not deemed an excuse. While frustrating, they don't signal an end to your good efforts or provide a reason to go off track completely.

Solutions to an injury might include the following:

- *Work around the problem*—Even when injured, you can usually do some form of exercise. For example, if you have an impact injury (stress fracture), you can hit the pool for some light swimming or aqua jogging (running with a floatation belt).
- *Get rehabilitated*—You will likely be prescribed a number of rehab exercises to do once your injury is diagnosed by a physiotherapist or doctor. These are time consuming, but they are essential to a fast and efficient recovery. Completing them daily will keep you focused and in a routine.

- *Focus on diet*—If your injury has significantly reduced your energy expenditure, closely check your diet to minimise weight gain from inactivity that can make it harder to get back into shape and good form. Making subtle adjustments of calorie restriction and reducing simple carbohydrate intake (sugars) will provide a feeling of control and damage limitation.

Solutions to an illness might include the following:

- *Eat well*—When battling an illness, you may feel deprived of energy and dehydrated. Eat small amounts often to prevent losing the valuable muscle you have built up during training and drink plenty of fluids to counter any ill effects of dehydration, such as cramps or something more serious.
- *Observe the above-the-neck rule*—If your symptoms are above the neck (blocked nose, cough, headache), it is generally accepted that you can continue with light exercise. If, however, your symptoms are below the neck, it is advised that you rest completely.

Lack of Motivation

This can be due to a number of factors—boredom, laziness, losing sight of your goals and lack of structure to your training or dietary programme. It can even occur for some people when they reach a goal and essentially think their work is done. Solutions to a lack of motivation might be to do the following:

- *Choose activities you enjoy*—If exercise is a chore rather than a pleasure, you will quite likely start to lose motivation. Find a class, sport or activity that you enjoy to keep your motivation high.
- *Find a training buddy*—Exercising with friends, family or colleagues is often more fun than training by yourself. Having made a commitment to meet them to exercise together, you're less likely to make excuses not to go.
- *Include variation*—If you do the same workout week in and week out, you most certainly will get bored and lose motivation. Rotate among several activities, classes and workout plans, selecting those relevant to your sport or end goal. This not only develops all-round fitness, but ensures you continue to challenge yourself and enjoy your exercise. Without variation, you will soon reach a plateau, whereby your results stagnate (fitness and weight). Break a plateau with a planned, progressive and varied routine.

Of course, other barriers to exercise exist—money, lack of knowledge, travel and more. Whatever your barrier is, be honest with yourself. Stop making excuses and start finding solutions. You may wish to use self-talk techniques, visualisation or simple brainstorming methods to help you to do this. Whatever method you choose, we hope the content of this book provides motivation and information to assist you on your journey towards your fitness goals.

Finally, let's consider a crucial point that is wholly pertinent as you are poised on the cusp of stepping into the unknown by ramping up your exercise routine. Since breaks in routine are almost inevitable, it makes sense to plan for them so they don't grow from a simple relapse into a major collapse. Common sense dictates that illness, work deadlines, family commitments and holidays may both expectedly and sometimes unexpectedly throw your programme off track. Accept that they happen. Rather than beating yourself up about it, reflect on the positive notion that you've already made changes and started some way down the road to a new you, and then move on. You can't stop the festive season, but a little forethought and the motivation to get straight back to your programme after a minor lapse will limit damage.

You should now feel armed with the requisite knowledge and self-belief to move off first base and take your training to the next level. As they say, there's no time like the present. So, what are you waiting for?

AT A GLANCE

- From the start, make sure your mindset is tuned up and ready for the journey ahead. You have the power to succeed. Write a mission statement and keep a few short positive thoughts in mind for when the going gets tough.

- Be prepared to work hard, harder than you ever have before, and understand that you need to do this consistently.

- Commit yourself mentally as well as physically to bringing about change. Use the SMART method to set goals that will help you guide your workout efforts and monitor your progress.

- Be honest with yourself regarding barriers and recognise that, with some careful forethought, you can overcome them fairly easily.

- Finally, accept that things will occasionally go wrong due to circumstances beyond your control. Steel yourself for these times and promise yourself that you will get straight back on the horse as soon as possible—and then ride it hard to your best-ever workout!

Fitness Assessments

2

If you fail to prepare, you prepare to fail! I'm sure you've heard that saying many times before, but do you apply it to your fitness and health? Of course you will notice some general and vague changes to your body and fitness if you keep moving in some way or another, but without assessment, a plan and structure to your workout, you will not see measurable, long-lasting results. So, the first step is to assess your current fitness level and body shape and then to take action by planning and executing the methods necessary for making improvements. Before we look at the actual assessments, let's get started by identifying body type.

BODY-TYPE IDENTIFICATION

The way your body responds to exercise is very much influenced by your genetics. In any given gym environment, you will see people of all shapes and sizes. Even those deemed very fit will have different body shapes and response patterns to exercise in the way that they develop muscle, burn fat and improve their cardiorespiratory fitness. Simply doing the same training as somebody whose body you admire and want for yourself may not work for you. Attaining your goal may require you to train specifically for your body type.

Of course, genetics determine that some people are naturally leaner and more responsive to exercise than others. Unfair, we know. There's not much you can do about that. With this in mind, you need to be realistic with your body-image goal and training targets. Can you really have the aerobic capacity of Paula Radcliffe or the physique of Elle Macpherson? The good news is that with the correct training for you and your body type, you can really push the boundaries of your genetic predisposition and be the best you can be (see chapter 1 and information about SMART to drive home the point that your goals must be realistic).

Body shapes have typically been classified as falling into one of three categories: *mesomorph, ectomorph* and *endomorph* (see figure 2.1). In reality, most people share characteristics from all three categories, but it is likely that you will identify with one category more than another. Each category has its own advantages and disadvantages in terms of health and fitness. Understanding these is the key to your success.

Read the following body-type descriptions and decide which best describes your body shape. Then reference the training responses and recommendations as well as disadvantages associated with your body type to help guide your exercise choice and training programme.

Mesomorph

The athletic physique for the mesomorph body type includes broad shoulders, narrow waist and hips, good muscular definition, low body fat and a reasonably fast metabolism. Mesomorph body types respond well to most types of training, especially resistance and body-shaping exercises, and sustain low body-fat levels. The disadvantages are that they can often become overtrained, so if you have the mesomorph body type, be mindful of incorporating rest days and lighter training sessions into your programme. Also, stagnation can easily occur if you are not challenged with a varying exercise routine. In this type, you can put on weight quickly when you stop training.

If you have a mesomorph body type it is recommended you do the following:

- Ensure all training methods are suitable and will elicit response and adaptation.
- Combine both major muscle and minor muscle group exercises into your routine.
- Utilise superset training to maximise effort during your workout time.
- Progress training regularly and vary it with regard to exercise modality, type and intensity.
- Favour steady-state and interval training over maximal sprints and lifts if your goal is to minimise muscle mass and use yoga, Pilates and lightweight, high-repetition circuit training to develop longer, leaner muscles.
- Allow adequate recovery between exercises and sets and between weight-training sessions if your goal is to maximise muscle mass. (This allows energy system regeneration in the first instance and muscle adaptation in the latter.)

Ectomorph

The athletic physique for the ectomorph body type includes narrow shoulders and hips, long, thin legs and arms, small bone structure and very little body fat. People with this type often look fragile. They find it easy to lose weight and keep it off. They are ideally suited to cardiovascular training due to their light frame and low body weight. The disadvantages are that they find it difficult to put on muscle and create a shapely physique, and they risk unhealthily low body-fat levels. They can also be prone to injury due to their fragile frame.

If you have an ectomorph body type it is recommended you do the following:

- Utilise split training whereby you train only one or two body parts with resistance exercises per session and aim to work each body part once per week.
- Take adequate rest between strength workouts to allow for muscle recovery and for optimal repair and adaptation (48-72 hours).
- Use heavy, basic power movements that target the deep muscle tissues.
- Use repetitions of 5 to 10 and perform 3 or 4 sets of each exercise.
- Keep cardiorespiratory activity to a minimum (maximum of three times per week) if your goal is to shape up and develop more muscle.
- Ensure good intake of protein and carbohydrate and increase calorie intake to maintain bodyweight and develop lean muscle.
- Enjoy a mix of running, cycling or rowing to minimise impact-based modalities if your goal is to maximise your genetic gift for aerobic exercise.
- Include adequate dietary calcium to further protect your bones, since some activities, such as running, can cause stress injuries for people with fragile frames.

Endomorph

The athletic physique for the endomorph body type includes wide hips and narrow shoulders that create a pear shape. People with this type have less muscle definition, uneven fat distribution (mostly accumulating in upper arms, bottom and thighs) with wide bone structure and a slower metabolism than those from other body types. Weight gain is easy and fat loss difficult for those in this category. Muscle definition tends to be hidden by fat. Endomorph body types respond well to power and strength training due to their natural strength. If they train and develop their muscles, then they can effectively increase their metabolic and fat-burning rates.

The disadvantages are that too much weight training in relation to aerobic activity can make them look bulky. They can also suffer joint problems if they carry too much body weight, as this puts stress on the joints. They also can find it more difficult to burn fat.

If you have an endomorph body type it is recommended you do the following:

- Include moderate-intensity, nonimpact cardiorespiratory exercise such as cycling and power walking on most, if not all, days of the week to achieve a leaner, lighter body shape.
- Ensure that cross training, which combines weights and cardiorespiratory training, is the basis of your training plan.
- Keep weights light, the repetition range between 10 and 25 and the recovery time short.
- Take extra care with your diet to eat regularly and reduce starchy and sugar-based carbohydrate opting instead for fibrous varieties and lean proteins (see chapter 3 for detailed dietary guidance and weight loss tips).

WEIGHT-LOSS TIP Try training and eating according to your body type for best results and body satisfaction. Trying to change your body shape will only lead to frustration and limited adaptation.

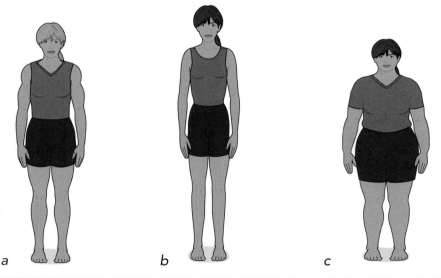

Figure 2.1 Body types: (a) mesomorph, (b) ectomorph and (c) endomorph.

WHAT IS YOUR FITNESS LEVEL?

Your fitness level is an indication of how well your body copes with a physical workload and recovers in a timely manner. Which of the following fitness levels currently applies to you?

- *Beginner*—You have little or virtually no gym or sporting experience or have just returned to training after a long break of 18 months or more.
- *Intermediate*—You have been training consistently for at least 9 months, undertaking 3 or 4 sessions per week with a combination of cardiorespiratory and resistance training exercises.
- *Advanced*—You have been training consistently for a long time (at least 18 months) with 4-plus sessions per week with a combination of cardiorespiratory and resistance exercises or sports-specific training.

We expect that most of you reading this book will fall between the intermediate and advanced levels of fitness described previously. This book takes your training to the next level with more progressive and advanced techniques and ideologies. Having identified your general fitness level, you can undertake specific assessments of the many different fitness components that come together to determine your overall fitness. This allows you to identify weaknesses and to select the exercises and training programmes that will help you improve.

FITNESS ASSESSMENTS

Now it's time to look more specifically at your fitness level by assessing your cardiorespiratory fitness, muscular strength, flexibility and body composition. A few reasons why fitness tests are necessary include the following:

- To assess your current fitness level
- To identify your fitness goals, interests and motivation for exercising
- To identify any areas of weakness that could be affecting your training progress and sports performance or even making you susceptible to injury
- To identify appropriate training options
- To establish methods to your track progress and evaluate programme success
- To adapt and progress your training programme at the correct rate

We know that some people dislike tests due to fear of the findings and the thought of being judged in some way. But fitness tests are a valuable tool in allowing you to assess your progress and plan effectively. Avoid comparing your results to those of others if you are sensitive and self-conscious; only compare them to your own previous markers. Remember, the tests are designed to help you! Select the tests most compatible with your fitness goals along with those considered baseline for general health and fitness assessment, which include the resting heart rate and maximal heart rate cardiorespiratory tests and the sit-and-reach flexibility test.

Cardiorespiratory Tests

Numerous tests for this category of fitness exist, with options to test your maximal and submaximal cardiorespiratory fitness. Some tests require sophisticated equipment and techniques (such as $\dot{V}O_2$max tests or lactate threshold tests), but we have selected simple tests that you can perform by yourself.

RESTING HEART RATE TEST

Monitoring resting heart rate (RHR) is a great way to measure improvements in cardiorespiratory fitness as, during a period of training, small changes in resting heart rate can reflect adaptation processes. As you get fitter, your resting heart rate should decrease because the heart becomes more efficient at pumping blood around the body. When you're at rest, more blood can be pumped around with each beat; therefore, fewer beats per minute (bpm) are needed. Heart rate can also be affected by ensuing illness, fatigue and overtraining, so regular monitoring can guide your rest and recovery requirements. This test is suitable for anyone of any fitness level.

Equipment

Heart rate monitor (optional)

How To

The measurement is ideally taken after 5 minutes of waking and whilst still lying in bed. To measure at any other time, first lie down for at least 10 minutes before taking a measurement. To take your heart rate manually using the palpation method, press two fingers (not your thumb) to either the carotid artery in your neck (see figure 2.2a) or the radial artery in your wrist (see figure 2.2b). Taking care not to press too hard, count the number of beats for a minute. If you have a heart rate monitor, attach it as per its instructions and take your reading. This will likely be the most accurate reading.

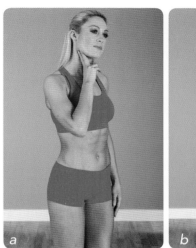
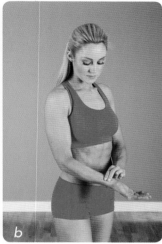

Figure 2.2   Taking your heart rate at the *(a)* carotid and *(b)* radial arteries.

Results

Note your resting heart rate and measure it regularly to monitor your fitness and physiological condition. An average resting heart rate for a woman is 75 bpm. RHR can fall to around 55 bpm in an elite female athlete.

Take Action!

A proven way to reduce your RHR is to become more aerobically fit so that you heart does less work to pump blood and oxygen around your body. See chapter 5: All In Aerobics, for a better understanding of this process and for workout examples that increase aerobic fitness and lower RHR.

MAXIMUM HEART RATE TEST

Your maximum heart rate (HRmax) is the highest number of heartbeats per minute when exercising maximally. It is best measured during a test in which the body is pushed to its limit. You can then use the percentage of your maximum heart rate as an indicator of exercise intensity and work to an exercise programme that uses percentage heart rates to set training loads. You can also calculate your maximum heart rate by subtracting your age from 220. This figure is only an estimate, but it's usually accurate to within 10 beats of your true maximum heart rate.

We've selected a treadmill test protocol for measuring your maximum heart rate. This test is suitable for intermediate and advanced exercisers, but not for those new to exercise or those with injuries or cardiorespiratory problems.

Equipment

Heart rate monitor with a chest strap (although you can take your pulse rate manually) or an exercise machine with a built-in heart rate monitor, such as a treadmill, elliptical machine or stationary bike.

How To

Warm up with 10 to 15 minutes of easy running on a treadmill. Then run for 3 minutes at a time, starting at 10 to 12 kilometres per hour and increasing your effort by 0.5 to 1.0 kilometres per hour until you can no longer continue. The test will likely last anywhere between 9 and 15 minutes, depending on the increments you choose and your fitness level. You may also wish to increase the gradient of the treadmill by 1 percent with each 3-minute interval. As soon as you stop, record your heart rate by either counting your pulse rate or noting the measurement on your monitor.

Results

The heart rate you record immediately after completing the test is your HRmax. Note that results may vary when tests are performed on different cardio machines and with different protocols, but progressive effort tests such as this one are more favourable than sprint tests, where the build-up of fatigue and lactic acid in the muscles may stop your effort before your heart rate reaches its maximum. Note that your maximum heart rate cannot increase through training. In fact, it actually decreases with age. However, with training, you can work selected percentages of your HRmax more efficiently.

Take Action!

Chapter 5: All In Aerobics will help you to improve the previously mentioned exercise efficiency. In particular, the fartlek and interval training methods encourage work at varying percentages of your HRmax.

SINGLE-EFFORT CARDIORESPIRATORY POWER TEST

This test looks at your cardiorespiratory output and performance over a single set distance or time period. It is suitable for intermediate and advanced exercisers who have a good understanding of pace and are familiar with the exercise machine and modality being used.

Equipment

Cardio exercise machine you are familiar with and confident using (e.g., rower, treadmill or stationary bike)

How To

On your chosen piece of equipment, work at maximum effort for a set period of time or distance (for example, 3-minute run or 5,000-metre row).

Results

Record your time or distance and note the protocol and settings you selected so you can compare them the next time you test. When you retest, use the same protocol, but aim to complete the distance faster or cover more distance in the set time.

Take Action!

Incorporate power training into your workout schedule to improve your single-effort cardiorespiratory power and, thus, performance in relevant sports such as those involving sprinting, jumping and throwing for a sustained period of time. Chapter 8: Power Up is packed with instructions for numerous power exercises, from plyometrics to Olympic lifts and sled sprints.

MULTIPLE-EFFORT CARDIORESPIRATORY POWER TEST

This test measures your cardiorespiratory power over a succession of intervals and indicates how well you can sustain your performance and effort. It is suitable for intermediate and advanced exercisers who have a good understanding of pace and are familiar with the cardio kit being used. It is especially suited to those who take part in interval-based sports, such as tennis, football and hockey.

Equipment

Cardio equipment you are familiar with (rower, treadmill or stationary bike)

How To

On your chosen piece of kit, work at maximum effort for a set period of time or distance and for a chosen number of repetitions (2 or more).

Results

Record your time or distance and note the protocol and settings you used so you can compare your results in the future. The next time you test, use the same protocol and aim to sustain your effort for a greater number of repetitions, cover more distance or record a faster time for the same number of repetitions.

Take Action!

Incorporate interval training into your workout routine to quickly make improvements in your multiple-effort cardio power and to simultaneously cut your workout time without compromising on results. Chapter 6: Go Anaerobic explains the science behind anaerobic training benefits (exercise in the absence of oxygen) and provides some great sample workouts.

SUBMAXIMAL CARDIORESPIRATORY FITNESS TEST

This test is a good guide to your general cardiorespiratory fitness. More specifically, it measures your performance, as distance covered, whilst working at a submaximal level of fitness. It is suitable for women at any fitness level who want a general assessment of their cardiorespiratory fitness.

Equipment

Cardio equipment you are familiar with (rower, treadmill or stationary bike) and a heart rate monitor (optional but ideal)

How To

Exercise continuously at a designated heart rate for a set time. For example, cycle for 20 minutes at a heart rate of 140 bpm or at RPE of 6/7 (see RPE scale on page 54 of chapter 4).

Results

Note the distance you covered and protocol you followed (i.e., heart rate and exercise time) so you can compare them the next time you test. Covering a greater exercise distance in the same time and at the same submaximal heart rate on subsequent attempts indicates an improvement in your submaximal cardiorespiratory fitness or general fitness.

Take Action!

Visit chapter 5: All In Aerobics and follow the continuous training and cross-training methods for improvements in your submaximal cardiorespiratory fitness.

THREE-MINUTE STEP TEST

This is a classic submaximal test that measures how efficiently your heartbeat returns to a resting rate after exercise. It is suitable for women at any fitness level who want a general assessment of their cardiorespiratory fitness.

Equipment

A step approximately 20 inches or 50 centimetres high, a stopwatch and a cadence tape or metronome set at 120 bpm (optional)

How To

Step up and down on the platform at a rate of 30 steps per minute (1 step every 2 seconds) for 3 minutes. Sit down immediately on completion of the test. After 10 seconds of rest, record your heartbeat over 1 minute by taking your pulse.

Results

Note your pulse rate as the beats per minute. For those interested in comparing their results with industry-standard results, table 2.1 shows the female norms.

Table 2.1   Three-Minute Step Test Norms for Women

Standard	Beats per minute (bpm)
Excellent	<73
Good	74–90
Average	91–100
Fair	101–114
Poor	<115

© John Shepherd, 2004, *Ultra fit: Your own personal trainer*, A&C Black, an imprint of Bloomsbury Publishing Plc.

Take Action!

You can improve your general cardiorespiratory fitness with a wide range of training methods, from steady-state cardio to interval training to fartlek training and more. See chapters 5 and 6 on aerobic and anaerobic training for additional information.

Muscular Strength Tests

Muscular strength tests fall into two categories—those that test for *maximal strength* (how much you can lift in one attempt) and those that test for *strength endurance* (your ability to perform a strength-orientated movement repeatedly until fatigue). The importance of each test to you will depend on your sport or exercise routine, but both can be useful measures of how you are progressing.

ONE-REPETITION MAX (1RM) TEST

The 1RM test assesses maximum strength and indicates how much weight you can lift in a single effort. Following a warm-up, use an exercise or lift that is appropriate to your training or sport. Common strength test exercises include squat, bench press, chest press and dead lift. The test provided here predicts your 1RM based on lighter-weight repetition numbers. It is suitable for those with basic and intermediate strength-training experience.

Equipment

Dumbbells, barbell, machine weights—basically, the equipment suitable for the lift or strength exercise you have chosen to test

How To

Select the exercise to use for the test and warm up with a light weight for 3 sets of 5 to 10 repetitions. Begin performing a 1-repetition individual lift at a weight below what you perceive to be your maximum. Rest for 5 minutes and repeat with a heavier weight. Continue to attempt single lifts with a 5-minute recovery until you fail your attempt. The last successful lift before failure is your actual 1RM. Ideally, you will reach your maximum weight on your third single attempt. Knowledge and experience of your lifting ability are important to getting an accurate result. If you attempt it too soon, you may not have activated your muscles effectively. If you repeat too many submaximal singles beforehand, you will be fatigued.

Results

Keep a record of your performance and the protocol used. Ideally, after a period of strength training, you will be able to lift a heavier weight when you retest. Your 1RM result is a useful measure for constructing your weight training programme. It will guide you on the percentage of this maximum to work at for your repetition exercises and, of course, will enable you to monitor your strength improvements over time.

Take Action!

To improve your maximal strength, check out both chapter 7: Going Strong and chapter 8: Power Up for information on the relevant training, as well as chapter 11 for sample workouts.

PUSH-UP TEST

The push-up test assesses strength endurance and is one of the most common tests for measuring it. However, the protocol doesn't have to be limited to the push-up. You may wish to replicate the test using other exercises that will test the strength endurance of other muscles in your body, such as a sit-up, squat or triceps dip. This test is suitable for women at any fitness level.

How To

Assume a military-style push-up position, touching the floor with only your hands and feet. If you have less upper body strength, bend your knees and place them on the floor as well (bent-knee style). To perform the push-up, position your hands under your shoulders with the elbows out (see figure 2.3a). Lower your chest as low as you can go without touching the ground (see figure 2.3b), and then push up to a straight-arm position, maintaining a strong, straight body position throughout. Do as many push-ups as

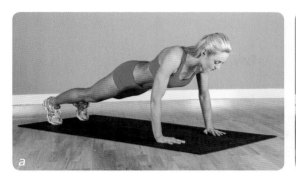 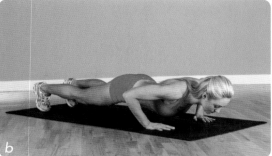

Figure 2.3   Push-up test.

possible until exhaustion, counting the repetitions as you go. Simply dip-
ping your chest to the ground whilst keeping your bum in the air does not
count as a repetition! Your body must remain straight for every counted
repetition, even if performed from your knees.

Results

Record the total number of push-ups performed so you can aim to improve
next time you test. Use table 2.2 to compare your results to a general standard of women aged 20 to 49 for the push-up exercise from your feet:

Table 2.2   **Push-Up Test Standards for Women**

	Age 20–29	Age 30–39	Age 40–49
Superior	>41	>39	>19
Excellent	28-41	23-29	16-19
Good	21-27	15-22	13-15
Fair	15-20	11-14	9-12
Poor	10-14	8-10	6-8
Very poor	<10	<8	<6

Adapted with permission from The Cooper Institute, Dallas, Texas, from *Physical Fitness Assessments and Norms
for Adults and Law Enforcement*. Available online at www.cooperinstitute.org.

Take Action!

Chapter 7: Going Strong challenges you to improve both your maximal
strength and strength endurance. You will find ways to improve your assessment results with a multitude of exercises and some workout examples. Some simply utilise your body weight, whilst others add resistance,
weight and even vibration.

Power Test

A power test measures your ability to move a load quickly so evaluating your strength and speed combined.

STANDING VERTICAL JUMP TEST

This classic power test assesses explosive power (pure power). If your sport or activity involves jumping (volleyball, basketball, netball, high jump), then this test is specifically relevant to you, but it's a valid measurement of muscular power for everyone.

How To

Stand next to a wall facing sideways. Chalk the hand closest to the wall and reach up, making sure to keep your feet flat on the floor (see figure 2.4a). Make a mark on the wall using your longest finger. Bending your knees at right angles (see figure 2.4b), jump as high as possible and make another mark with your hand (see figure 2.4c). Measure the distance between the two marks. Repeat a total of three times, again making sure to fully recover between efforts. Take your best score of the three trials.

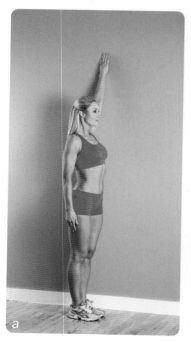 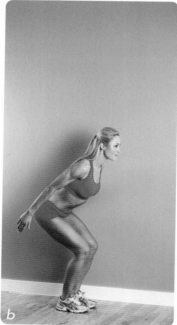 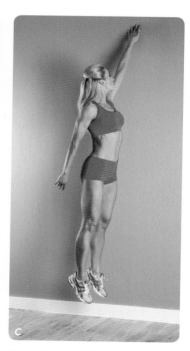

Figure 2.4   Standing vertical jump test.

Results

Table 2.3 provides the female standards with which you can compare your performance.

Table 2.3 Vertical Jump Test Standards for Women

Standard	Height
Excellent	>53 cm
Good	41-52 cm
Average	30-40 cm
Needs improvement	<29 cm

Adapted, by permission, from E.P. Roetert and T.S. Ellenbecker, 2007, *Complete conditioning for tennis* (Champaign, IL: Human Kinetics), 32.

Take Action!

To improve your results, include Olympic lifts and box jumps in your weekly training routine. Chapter 11 provides sample workouts for you to try.

Flexibility Test

Flexibility tests usually involve the linear measurement of distances between your body parts or from an external object. Overall flexibility can be difficult to assess, as most of us have greater flexibility in one area or side of our body than another. It is therefore important to measure flexibility through several tests across different body parts. Here we provide an example of one of the most common tests.

SIT-AND-REACH TEST

The sit-and-reach test has long been used as a standard measure of flexibility. It is particularly important for anyone taking part in sport and exercise involving sprinting and jumping, which put the hamstrings under extra stress. This test is suitable for anyone who does not have any spinal disc problems (in that case, avoid flexing the spine).

Equipment

Use a ruler and a step (the bottom of a staircase or a stand-alone box roughly the height of your foot length).

How To

Warm up with some light cardio and dynamic stretches (see chapter 4: Warming Up and Cooling Down). Sit on a flat surface, with the legs extended in front of your body, toes pointing up and feet slightly apart. Brace the soles of your feet against the base of the step (see figure 2.5a). Place the ruler on the top of the step and one hand on top of the other, and then reach slowly forward, keeping your back flat and your head in line with your body (see figure 2.5b). Hold the stretch for a couple of seconds, and then measure the distance you have reached. If you do not reach the step, measure the distance between the point you reached and the step; this is a negative measurement score.

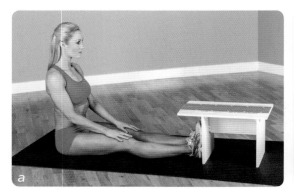
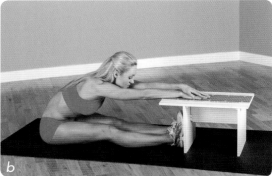

Figure 2.5   Sit-and-reach test.

Results

Record your distance to compare next time. For women, more than 8 centimetres is considered an excellent score, 5 to 8 centimetres is average and less than 2 centimetres is poor.

Take Action!

To improve your flexibility scores, incorporate various forms of stretching into your workout plan. Chapter 4: Warming Up and Cooling Down will guide you on which type of stretches to perform and when to perform them, as well as every stretch exercise needed for improving your flexibility in a desired muscle. To improve your hamstring flexibility and, therefore, the results in this test, look for stretches indicated for hamstrings.

Body Composition Tests

Body composition describes the different components and tissue types that make up your body weight, including lean tissues (muscle, bone and organs), which are metabolically active, and fat (adipose), which is not.

Standard body-weight scales will provide you with a measure of total body weight, but they will not determine the lean-to-fat ratio of that weight or, in other words, how much of that weight is muscle and how much is fat. Typically when you begin or advance your exercise routine, you will increase your muscle mass and, consequently, your weight, as the same volume of muscle weighs more than that of fat! This can be disheartening when you've been putting in the gym time to lose weight. Rest assured, though, this increase in muscle weight actually translates to a slimmer, stronger, leaner you if you adhere to consistent exercise and good nutrition. So, body composition tests are more reflective of your progress.

Body composition tests can be a great measure of your progress both in terms of performance and aesthetics, but it is important not to obsess over your results. Remember that this is just one component of your training progress. A low level of body fat is related to improved sporting performance, but it is also sport dependent. If your body fat becomes extremely low, you risk injury, decreased performance and health issues.

Now that we've raised the preoccupation warning, let's look at testing methods. Many different methods exist for assessing your body fat and lean mass percentages, each with different levels of accuracy. The key is to be as consistent as possible with the protocol of your choice so that differences over time reflect changes in your body rather than in your measurement practice. One way to ensure this is to be tested by the same person, with same equipment and at the same time of day each time. The following methods are the best and most practical tests for you to perform on your own.

BODY MASS INDEX (BMI) TEST

This method for estimating body fat percentage is based on simple weight and height measurements. Although it is an indirect measurement, it can be a reliable indicator of body fat in the average person. However, it tends to be less accurate for athletes who display a high BMI. This is due to their high levels of muscle mass, which weighs more than fat. It's actually possible for someone who is very lean and muscled to achieve an 'overweight' BMI score, as if she had a high body-fat percentage! Although this test is suitable for anyone, be aware that results for highly trained athletes may not be accurate.

Equipment

Weighing scales, measure tape and calculator

How To

Measure your height and your weight, divide your weight in kilograms by your height in metres squared, and then compare your result to the figures in the BMI chart in the following section. For example, if you weigh 65 kilograms and are 1.7 metres tall, your BMI would be:
65 ÷ (1.7 × 1.7 [=2.89]) = 22

Results

Interpret your result using table 2.4:

Table 2.4   BMI Results for Women

	BMI
Underweight	<18.5
Normal weight	18.5–24.9
Overweight	25–30
Obese	>30

Source: National Health Service, NHS Choices. Available: www.nhs.uk/livewell/loseweight/pages/bodymassindex.aspx [June 17, 2013].

Take Action!

If your BMI falls outside of the normal weight range, it may be time for you to take action. If you are underweight, consider whether you are refuelling from your workouts with enough food and the right composition of macronutrients. Chapter 3: Nutrition Matters provides advice on meals and snacks for your exercise type, with specific quantities of macronutrients suited to your body weight. You may also benefit from increasing your lean muscle mass. Chapter 7: Going Strong provides exercises and protocols to help you. Remember that the BMI test is not the most accurate measure for athletes, especially if they are particularly muscular. If you are an Olympic weightlifter, rower or rugby player with a high muscle mass, then this test may interpret your measures as obese when clearly you are not. In this case, a fat percentage test is more accurate. If, however, you are overweight or obese, consider losing weight to improve your overall health and sporting performance. Incorporating a variety of exercises—aerobic, anaerobic and strength training—and focusing on healthy eating will put you on course to improve your BMI result.

WAIST-TO-HIP RATIO TEST

Like the BMI test, the waist-to-hip ratio test indicates whether your body is within acceptable body-fat levels. Fat is stored beneath the skin and also around the vital organs with research showing that fat around the abdomen presents a greater risk to health than that held on the hips and thighs. Excess fat around the middle is linked to increases likelihood of developing type 2 diabetes and heart problems. Be aware, though, that if you have a very athletic physique with narrow hips, the test may suggest that you are too lean. This test is suitable for anyone of any fitness level.

Equipment

Measure tape and calculator

How To

Measure your waist at the point of maximum girth (above your hip bone) and your hips at the point where your bottom protrudes the most. Then simply divide your waist measurement by your hip measurement in centimetres (or inches), and record and compare your results to the following standards guide.

WEIGHT-LOSS TIP

The most effective way to lose weight around your midsection is not to do hundreds of sit-ups but to control your insulin levels by regularly eating (every 2 to 4 hours) carbohydrate low on the glycaemic index combined with good fat and lean protein. Insulin spikes following consumption of sugary foods have been linked to abdominal fat, so follow this advice to help shift those midsection pounds!

Results

Interpret your results using table 2.5:

Table 2.5   Waist-to-Hip Ratio Standards for Women

	Age 20-29	Age 30-39	Age 40-49
Low risk	<0.71	<0.72	<0.73
Moderate risk	0.71–0.77	0.72-0.78	0.73-0.79
High risk	0.78–0.82	0.79-0.84	0.80-0.87
Very high risk	>0.82	>0.84	>0.87

Adapted, by permission, from V.H. Heyward and D.R. Wagner, 2004, *Applied body composition assessment*, 2nd ed. (Champaign, IL: Human Kinetics), 78.

Take Action!

If your value is either average or high, it is deemed unacceptable. You must take action to reduce the size of your stomach, as this is the most dangerous place to store fat in terms of the risk of coronary heart disease. Moreover, a fat waist is not going to help your mobility or sporting performance! Your diet is largely responsible for the size of your waist, so make a priority to clean it up. Visit chapter 3: Nutrition Matters for meal suggestions and tips for weight loss.

BIOELECTRICAL IMPEDANCE ANALYSIS (BIA) BODY-FAT TEST

This method sends a low level of safe, electrical current through the body. The current travels at a different rate through the various body tissues, which then allows a calculation of fat mass and lean (fat-free) mass. The current will pass easily through muscle tissue, but travels slowly through the fat tissue. The resistance it experiences as it hits the fat tissue is called *bioelectrical impedance.* This feature is common in many digital weighing scales, such as Tanita or Omron. With the addition of information on your height, gender and weight, these scales can then compute your body-fat percentage. Readings can be affected by your hydration levels, food intake and skin temperature, amongst other factors, but you will generate useful results if you use the scales under similar conditions each time. This test is suitable for anyone of any fitness level.

WEIGHT-LOSS TIP Although your BMI and waist-to-hip ratio measures are great for assessing your progress towards your weight-loss goals, a reduction in these measures can sometimes indicate an undesired loss in valuable muscle tissue as well as fat tissue. Look at your body-fat percentage as a more useful indicator that you are becoming leaner, not just smaller!

Equipment

Digital scales with a BIA feature

How To

Follow the instructions on your scales to obtain a digital reading of your body-fat percentage.

Results

Record your result and observe the most commonly used body-fat chart in table 2.6 to interpret your score.

Table 2.6 ACE Body-Fat Percentage for Women

	Body fat
Essential fat	10–13%
Athletes	14–20%
Fitness	21–24%
Average	25–31%
Obese	32%+

© 2010 American Council on Exercise

Take Action!

If your results indicate that your body-fat level is not desirable or suitable for your sport or activity, then you need to take action. The most effective way to lose body fat is through dietary changes (see chapter 3: Nutrition Matters) and a combination of workouts designed to build muscle mass (see chapter 7: Going Strong) and those that are high in intensity (see chapter 6: Go Anaerobic and chapter 8: Power Up). This is because increased muscle mass increases your metabolic rate throughout the day, making you a greater fat-burning machine. High-intensity training increases your excess postexercise oxygen consumption (EPOC) so you continue to burn fat at a greater rate during the hours following exercise (see chapter 7: Going Strong).

Another way to learn your fat percentage is the skinfold thickness measurement test. This common test for body fat, performed by a personal trainer or physiologist, can be up to 98 percent accurate if the tester is skilled. The test estimates your percentage of body fat by measuring skinfold thickness at specific locations on your body. As the test requires the assistance of a professional, we have not included the protocol here. However, if your gym, training facility or physician has the tools and someone available to assist you, you may want to use this measure.

Your fitness tests should be performed regularly throughout the year, usually every 6 to 8 weeks, or at the completion of each training cycle (if you are indeed working in cycles). Your body composition tests can be performed at the same time or even at weekly intervals if you are making significant dietary changes or if this practice helps you to stay on track. However, be advised that weekly body composition measurements can vary quite considerably depending on the phase of your menstrual cycle.

Progress and rate of change and development will vary from person to person and between the different fitness measures, but aim for a gradual and steady rate of improvement with results that can be sustained over the long term. You will face plateaus, but the training advice and workouts in this book should give you new stimulus and information to break through them. Remember, quick-fix attempts bring about fast but unsustainable results! Assess, train and eat correctly for your body type and training goals, and then retest.

AT A GLANCE

- Assessing your fitness level is important for obtaining current fitness measures, identifying goals and motivations for exercising, identifying areas of weakness, selecting appropriate training options and for progressing your programme at the correct rate.
- At the most general level, fitness can be assessed by identifying whether you are a beginner, intermediate or advanced exerciser.
- Body-type identification can be useful for determining the best exercise solutions for you, as your genetics play a big factor in your body shape and subsequently how you will respond to exercise. Body types can be classified as *mesomorph* (muscular and square), *ectomorph* (long and lean) or *endomorph* (wide hips and narrow shoulders).
- More specific fitness tests include those for cardiorespiratory fitness and strength.
- Cardiorespiratory abilities can be tested by (a) resting heart rate, (b) maximum heart rate, (c) single-effort cardiorespiratory power, (d) multieffort cardiorespiratory power and (e) submaximal cardiorespiratory fitness, as well as (f) with a general aerobic fitness test.
- Strength can be assessed through tests for maximal strength (one-repetition max tests) or strength endurance (e.g., push-up test).
- Power can be tested with the standing vertical jump test and improved with Olympic lifts and plyometric exercises such as box jumping.
- Flexibility is most commonly assessed with a sit-and-reach test but other body parts could be tested to identify imbalances.
- Body composition assessments include BMI tests, waist-to-hip ratio tests, and bioelectrical impedance tests for measuring body-fat percentage.

3

Nutrition Matters

Good nutrition is fundamental to getting the best results from your workout and achieving your goals, whether they are related to performance, fitness or aesthetics. Despite this, keen exercisers and athletes commonly put 100 percent effort into their workouts only to let themselves down with a poor understanding and execution of their diet.

This chapter covers essential information, tips and meal plans to help you fuel and re-fuel your body for optimal results. It also addresses the important area of hydration, including sports drinks and the minefield subject of supplements.

PREWORKOUT FUEL

Eating the right food at the right time before your workout is essential for optimal energy, performance, comfort and well-being. Get it wrong, and you'll sell yourself short or, worse still, suffer hunger at one extreme and indigestion at the other! In addition to being easily digestible, your pre-workout foods and fluids should satisfy your hunger, restock carbohydrate stores that may have become depleted following a previous workout or overnight fast, hydrate or rehydrate your body, optimise performance and prepare your body for rapid recovery post exercise.

When To Eat?

Ideally, you should eat 2 to 4 hours before you begin to exercise. This allows your body enough time to digest the food. Provided you eat the right food, you will still have energy by the time you begin.

A common mistake is to eat a meal high in carbohydrate too close to exercise. This leaves you feeling uncomfortable, nauseated and possibly weak, as your blood supply is directed to your digestive organs instead of your muscles. For example, taking in carbohydrate only 1 hour before exercise may cause an insulin response that leads to hypoglycaemia (low blood sugar)

FUEL AND EARLY-MORNING WORKOUTS

If you favour an early-morning workout, avoid exercising on an empty stomach. Though this depends on the quality of your diet overall and some evidence exists that this practice will help you to lose weight (as carbohydrate stores are depleted in the morning and your body therefore relies on fat mobilisation), it's not our recommendation. Exercising with low blood glucose levels can induce early fatigue, which could increase injury risk and also reduces overall calorie burn. You will likely overeat after the session as your appetite and your body's need for fuel go into overdrive. If your goal is weight loss, your daily energy balance and composition of what you eat will matter more than a fasted workout. If you simply can't face eating early in the morning, experiment with different food options until you find something you can tolerate, even if it is a liquid meal such as a sports drink, protein shake, smoothie or juice that contains fast-release protein or high-glycaemic carbohydrate.

during the first few minutes of exercise. If you need a preworkout boost of energy or if you are exercising early in the day, have a snack of something easy to digest, such as a banana or a handful of berries. In this case, you can snack 10 minutes before you exercise without adverse effects. You will not experience hypoglycaemia as there is simply not enough time for your body to respond by pumping out insulin. By the time exercise begins, the body immediately starts to downregulate its need for insulin. The following section lists examples of suitable preworkout meals and snacks.

What to Eat?

It is easy to choose good preworkout foods according to their macronutrient category, so we will look at carbohydrate, protein and fat, plus fibre in turn to help you make the best selections.

The majority of calories in your preworkout meal, around 60 to 70 percent, should come from carbohydrate. The carbohydrate will raise your blood glucose levels, boost muscle and liver glycogen levels and aid performance, particularly endurance performance. If chosen correctly, the advantage of carbohydrate is that it is digested fairly quickly. Choose foods with carbohydrate types that have a low glycaemic index (GI) and therefore release their energy slowly (see table 3.1 for a list of popular foods and their GI). All ingested carbohydrate releases sugar, which triggers your pancreas to release the hormone insulin. This results in a rapid decrease in the body's

Table 3.1   GI for Popular Foods

Low GI foods	Moderate GI foods	High GI foods
Fruit (apples, pears, plums, cherries, peaches, grapefruit)	Fruit (oranges, grapes, kiwi, berries, mango)	Fruit (watermelon, papaya, pineapple, bananas) and dried fruit (raisins, dates, prunes)
Vegetables (broccoli, green beans, asparagus, spinach)	Vegetables (sweet potatoes, peas, carrots, bell peppers)	Vegetables (baked potatoes, beets/beetroot, parsnips)
Grains (barley, bulgar, rye)	Grains (white rice, brown rice, wild rice, basmati rice, couscous)	Grains (instant white rice, millet)
Breads (wholegrain pumpernickel)	Breads (whole-wheat, pita, sourdough)	Breads (white bread, bagels)
Cereals (All-Bran)	Cereals (oatmeal, Special K and Grape Nuts)	Cereals (cornflakes, Rice Krispies, puffed wheat)
Snacks (peanuts, macadamias, almonds, walnuts, Brazil)	Snacks (rye crisp breads, popcorn, potato chips/ crisps)	Snacks (rice cakes, corn chips, pretzels, crackers, chocolate, sweets/candy, biscuits, pancakes)
Meat, fish, eggs	White or whole-wheat pasta	Honey and sweetened preserves (jam)
Cheese, milk (cow and soy), plain yogurt		
Beans (lentils, navy, kidney, soy, black, chickpeas)		
Oils (olive, walnut, sunflower)		

blood sugar level, followed shortly by increased hunger. Different sources of carbohydrate release their sugar at different rates, and the GI indicates the speed at which a food releases its sugar. Good examples of low-GI carbohydrates include wholegrain breads, porridge, beans and lentils. As a general rule, the earlier you eat before a workout, the lower the food you choose should be on the glycaemic index.

You should also add some protein to your preworkout meal to further slow the release of the carbohydrate and delay the onset of fatigue. Complete proteins (those that contain all the essential amino acids your body needs) are a good choice. These include eggs, lean meat (chicken and turkey) and fish. You can add incomplete proteins (those that contain some but not all of the essential amino acids), which are often more convenient and readily available. These include nuts, beans, lentils and yogurt. Three essential amino acids in particular, known as branched-chain amino acids (BCAA), have been found to benefit performance when taken before aerobic exercise. Other research has shown that combining these BCAA with carbohydrate before strenuous exercise stimulates protein synthesis afterwards, improving your speed of recovery. Whole eggs are a good source of BCAA; you can also use supplements.

Fatty foods (fried food especially) delay digestion and can cause discomfort. In particular, fat remains in the stomach for a long time, often pulling blood there to help aid digestion, which can cause abdominal cramping of the stomach and deprive the muscles of the blood for exercise. Avoid meats, fries, nuts and candy bars before your workout.

Though high-fibre foods have a low GI and are a great part of a general daily diet, they may be too effective as a pre-exercise meal. The fibre in some foods can be so dense that it sits in your gut for several hours, soaking up fluids and swelling. Keep your preworkout meal low in fibre to avoid unnecessary discomfort.

Low-fat dairy is an acceptable food choice for some people before a workout. However, those who suffer from lactose intolerance, which can lead to lethargy, acid build-up, bloating, gas and burping, should eliminate dairy to avoid feeling discomfort and being slowed down during their workout.

Preworkout Meal and Snack Suggestions

Some recommended meals for 2 to 4 hours pre exercise include the following:

- *Porridge oats made with water, added berries and ground flaxseeds*—Oats provide a great slow release of energy whilst the berries provide antioxidant vitamins. Flaxseeds are high in omega-3s, and they lower the GI of the meal further.

- *Broth-based soup with chicken and soft vegetables*—Lean protein and easily digestible vegetables are a great combination of slow-release carbohydrate and protein. As an added bonus, the broth provides fluid for hydration.

- *Sweet potato with tuna*—Sweet potato has a lower GI value than a regular potato and is packed with vitamins, whilst the tuna provides a great protein addition.

- *Boiled egg and fresh fruit*—Eggs are loaded with protein and are easily digested by most people. Combine with a banana or melon which are an easily digestible fruit choice.

- *Oatcakes with cottage cheese*—Oatcakes are a light snack that, when combined with 100 grams plus of cottage cheese, feel quite substantial and satisfying. Cottage cheese is high in protein and low in fat. Combine it with pineapple chunks or herbs for added flavour.

- *Baby food*—This may sound like an odd choice for an adult, but it is easily sourced and digested by the human gut at any age. Good choices are those with fruits or vegetables. Combine them with chopped meats such as turkey, fish or chicken.

- *Meal-replacement bars*—Though these are our least recommended option for added protein, due to being highly processed, they can be a valuable go-to option when real food is not readily available, and they can be purchased almost everywhere and carried in your bag. Though most are primarily carbohydrate based, some also contain protein to slow the glycaemic reaction and add some BCAA to the meal. However, they can be dry, and they may draw fluids from your body into the gut to assist with digestion, leaving you dehydrated, so you must drink lots of water with them.

- *Blended low-fibre fruit, fruit juice and protein powder*—Combining easily digested carbohydrate—again with protein, including BCAA—helps the body release energy slowly. Some people can stomach this liquid formula more easily than whole foods. Add some low-fat yogurt if you want to create a more substantial meal.

Also, as mentioned in the previous section, you can have a snack 10 minutes before exercise. Select a carbohydrate source with a moderate to high GI for instant energy. Good choices include bananas, dried fruit and cereal bars. However, be careful of too much sugar as this may cause a rebound drop in blood glucose levels (hypoglycaemia) during your workout, leading to light-headedness, nausea and early fatigue. As a guide, limit the amount of sugar in your preworkout snack to fewer than 25 grams (one medium banana contains approximately 18 g of sugar).

Some recommended snacks for 10 minutes before exercise include the following:

- *Dried fruit*—A small serving (about 30 grams) of dried fruit such as raisins provides instant energy.

- *Natural yogurt with honey*—Honey is a natural sugar with a high GI value for instant energy. Combine with natural yogurt for a light snack (provided you do not suffer adverse effects from dairy) or simply add a spoonful to warm water for a liquid snack.

- *Banana*—This fruit has a high GI value for instant energy and contains potassium to help balance your electrolytes. Sometimes just half or a few mouthfuls can be enough to provide an energy boost without making you feel too full.

- *Berries*—Sweet and easily digested, a handful of berries such as raspberries, blueberries or strawberries are ideal.

- *Mini pancakes*—Commercially available and light and easily digested for a preworkout energy boost, one to three pancakes do the job! Even better if you can make your own and add berries to the mix!

- *Jaffa cakes*—These are also light and easily digested before training. They are calorific if too many are eaten (they are very tasty!) so moderate your intake to three or four depending on your size and energy needs.

- *Sports drink or gel*—Consuming 100 to 200 calories from a drink or gel with around 200 millilitres of water provides an effective energy boost for those who can't stomach whole foods.

How Much to Eat?

The number of calories you consume in your preworkout meal (and preworkout snack) will depend on the timing of your meal, the length and intensity of your workout and your body size. So you should consume more calories the larger you are, the sooner you eat before your workout and the longer or more intense your workout will be. The closer you are to your workout, the less you should eat. The following guide is for calorie consumption according to when you choose to eat your preworkout meal or snack:

WEIGHT-LOSS TIP If your workout goal is weight loss, skip the last-minute preworkout snack. The carbohydrate boost this provides delays fat burning, as your body works to metabolise the carbohydrate as the primary fuel. But have your preworkout meal at least two hours before exercise rather than up to four hours, with choices from our selection to ensure sufficient energy for your workout.

- *4 hours pre workout*: 400 to 500 calories
- *2 hours pre workout*: 200 to 400 calories
- *10 minutes pre workout*: 100 to 200 calories (often suitable as liquid)

POSTWORKOUT FUEL

You've just pushed out your final repetition or powered through the last few gruelling minutes of that spin class. You're now ready for some essential recovery nutrition to get the best results from your training and remain consistent across all workouts.

Your postworkout fuelling begins with a snack during the all-important 30-minute window immediately after exercise, when your body is at its most receptive to the nutrients you consume, and then continues with a meal 2 to 4 hours post exercise. The goals during this 30-minute window are to replace your muscles' carbohydrate stores and provide protein to repair the naturally occurring muscle damage that takes place during exercise, especially when you have performed strength and power work. It is also vitally important you rehydrate and replace your body's electrolytes. Your refuelling goal for 2 to 4 hours post workout is complete nutrition that focuses on macronutrient recovery, primarily that of carbohydrate and protein. After 4 hours, your diet should reflect your general needs as an endurance- or strength-based athlete or general exerciser.

The following sections address postworkout macronutrient needs during the 30-minute window and the 2 to 4 hours after exercise, as well as your hydration and electrolyte requirements.

30-Minute Window

Within 30 minutes after exercise, choose carbohydrates with a high GI, such as sports drinks containing glucose (isotonic or hypertonic), for quick replacement of muscle glycogen. This liquid meal begins the rehydration process, and it is easier to stomach than whole foods. If you can stomach whole foods, then your choices will be similar to the 10-minute preworkout snacks identified earlier, as they contain readily available glucose.

During an intense 1-hour workout, it's possible to use 30 grams (1 oz) of muscle protein for fuel. Protein sources, especially those rich in BCAA, should therefore be taken during this 30-minute window at a carbohydrate-to-protein ratio of around 4:1 after an aerobic endurance training session and 2:1 after a resistance training or anaerobic session. Research indicates that a good carbohydrate–protein combination post workout leads to a significantly greater muscle glycogen replacement as well as greater strength development compared to ingesting carbohydrate alone. Opt for complete protein sources such as egg whites or whey protein powder in a recovery drink as they contain all the essential amino acids your body needs for the purpose of resynthesis of muscle protein and they can be easily digested immediately post workout. An intense workout, especially if strength and power based, also causes some muscle cell damage to occur. This process, as mentioned before, is necessary for muscle rebuilding and development, but it relies on adequate replacement of BCAA, the building blocks for repair. This is present most notably in eggs and through supplementation.

2 to 4 Hours After the Workout

At this stage, focus on carbohydrate replenishment if you have performed an endurance workout. However, the type of carbohydrate you consume should contain more starches, which have a high glycaemic load (GL). The GL is a measure of how fast the food's sugar gets into the blood together with how much carbohydrate is delivered. Good food choices include sweet potato; grains such as rice, bread and cereal; as well as dried fruits, such as raisins. Your appetite should serve as a guide as to how much to eat, though eat slowly and chew food thoroughly so your brain receives this signal that your stomach is full. This usually takes about 20 minutes. Carbohydrate intake at this stage is less important for those having completed strength-based workouts and those focused on weight loss. Once you have adequately replenished your muscle glycogen levels, your carbohydrate requirements go down, and the type you need to consume changes from high-GI and high-GL foods to low-GI fruits and vegetables containing more fibre and micronutrients. Some examples of the many low-GI fruits and vegetables include apples, pears and berries for fruit choices and broccoli, cabbage, cauliflower and sprouts as your vegetable choices. Our general carbohydrate recommendations for those performing low- to moderate-intensity exercise are 5 to 7 grams per kilogram per day and for those performing high-intensity exercise are 7 to 12 grams per kilogram per day.

Your body still requires amino acids for resynthesis of muscle protein two to four hours post workout as well as for general maintenance of physiological structures such as the nervous system, so meals should contain adequate protein by way of whole foods. Animal products are great choices as they are complete proteins. Fish, egg whites and lean meats such as turkey and chicken breast are ideal. These proteins also lower the GI of the carbohydrate foods eaten at the same time, which helps control blood sugar levels. As an athlete or committed exerciser, you should consume more protein throughout the day than a sedentary or less active person due to your enhanced needs for essential amino acids to repair damaged muscle tissue. However, how much you need depends on your body weight, particularly your muscle mass, your training volume and the intensity of your training. Heavy lifting, sprint and power training also increase your protein requirements. We recommend protein intakes of 1.2 to 1.4 grams per kilogram per day for athletes participating in aerobic and endurance exercise and 1.6 to 1.8 grams per kilogram per day for those involved in anaerobic and strength-based activities. Again, animal products are the best sources of protein. Vegetarians may opt for plant-based sources such as grains and beans, with quinoa being a particularly good choice as it contains the highest number of essential amino acids. However, the quantity of these you will need to eat to get adequate daily protein is considerably

WEIGHT-LOSS TIP If your goal is weight loss, don't make the mistake of removing fat from your diet. Eating good fats actually helps your body to mobilise and metabolise more fat. Fat also has a high satiety factor, helping you to feel full for longer. Low-fat diets are certainly not recommended for active women, as they decrease energy and nutrient intake and reduce exercise performance. We do however advise you to reduce saturated fats (bad fats) from your diet, those found in fatty meats and whole dairy foods, as well as trans fats, sometimes called partially hydrogenated oil, found in many processed foods and ready meals, but overall, fat is not the enemy when it comes to weight loss!

higher, so you may fall short of consuming all the essential amino acids. Therefore, it may be advisable for vegetarian athletes to use protein supplementation.

Though ingesting fat is not essential during the 30-minute window post workout, the intake of good fats forms a valuable part of your daily diet and helps with general recovery and well-being. The most desirable fats are omega-3 fatty acids, as they have been found to reduce inflammation, a common and persistent problem for athletes, by lowering the ratio of omega-6 to omega-3 fatty acids (which should be approximately 2:1). In today's society, we consume far more omega-6 than this, mostly through readily available packaged foods, vegetable oils and grain products, so it is important to redress the balance. Good sources of omega-3s include oily fish (salmon, mackerel, and tuna), leafy vegetables, walnuts, omega-3-enriched eggs, fish oils and flaxseed oil supplements.

Finally, it's quite likely you will be slightly dehydrated after your workout. You will need to drink to replace the fluids lost from sweating. How much fluid you lose depends on your preworkout hydration, fluid consumed during your workout as well as the duration and intensity of your workout. Consider also that environmental factors such as heat and humidity also increase your sweat rate and volume. You can calculate your fluid loss by weighing yourself before and then immediately after your workout. A 1-kilogram loss is roughly equivalent to 1 litre of water (1 pound is approximately 0.5 litres). Use this measure to calculate the amount of fluid you need to drink to rehydrate. You don't need to drink it all in one go, and this would likely be difficult and uncomfortable, but plan to continue this hydration process over the next few hours as your body's hydration needs continue, perhaps even consuming 150 percent of what your weight indicates you have lost to be certain of complete rehydration. During exercise, your body also loses a small amount of electrolytes, mainly sodium, through sweat. These losses are most critical in endurance events and in extreme heat. You can replace any lost electrolytes with natural foods consumed post workout, especially with fruit, which contains most of the electrolytes lost during exercise. Sodium can be replaced by consuming a recovery sports drink, adding a few pinches of salt to fruit juice or eating a salty snack such as pretzels. See the next section for more information on general fluid intake.

FLUID

Your body is 65 to 75 percent water, so it's vitally important you hydrate, rehydrate and avoid dehydration throughout the day. Water performs the general body functions of regulating temperature through sweating, acting as a medium for chemical reactions, eliminating waste products and toxins, lubricating the digestive track and providing a carrier for blood cells amongst others. Water is quite simply the most essential part of our diet.

The most common recommendation for hydration is 2 litres per day (or around 6 to 8 glasses), but your need may vary from that of others, depending on your activity, body size and food consumption. For general daily hydration, we personally prescribe 1 millilitre per calorie consumed and advise you to be aware of specific indicators of your hydration as follows:

- *Thirst*—By the time you're thirsty, you are already dehydrated. Don't wait until you reach this stage before reaching for a drink.
- *Urine colour and quantity*—Your urine should be relatively clear, fairly substantial in volume and odourless. Dark, smelly or scant (merely a trickle) urine output suggests that undiluted toxins and waste products have built up. Please note, however, some nutrition supplements can also lead to darker colour urine, so keep this in mind when assessing your hydration level.
- *Mouth moisture*—A dry mouth is often a sign of dehydration and is one of the first signs of its onset.
- *Headache*—This is a common symptom of dehydration and a sign that you need to drink more water.
- *Muscle cramps*—These involuntary contractions of the muscle are often associated with dehydration and the associated electrolyte disruption.
- *Elevated heart rate*—When you are dehydrated, you have either less fluid in your blood or a lower blood volume. This means your body requires more effort to circulate blood. Your heart therefore has to beat more often, raising your heart rate.

THE LOWDOWN ON SPORTS DRINKS

With so many sports drinks on the market and extensive advertising about their benefits, it can become confusing to select one and to understand when is best to drink it. The first decision, however, should be whether you actually need one at all.

Many gym enthusiasts, especially those new to exercise, consume a sports drink only to ingest calories in excess of those being expended, prevent fat mobilisation due to the additional carbohydrate consumed and sometimes feel sick from high sugar levels. The truth is that if you are exercising continuously or for weight-loss purposes for less than 60 minutes, and if you've eaten properly in the hours leading up to your workout, then it's best to simply drink water. A sports drink is only a useful hydration method if you exceed 60 minutes of exercise, if you are focused on performance over weight loss or if you've not eaten properly before a workout, especially if you're performing an early-morning workout and you can't stomach whole foods.

Three types of sports drink exist, all of which contain various levels of fluid, electrolytes and carbohydrate. The following section describes them and helps you decide if any are suitable for your workout needs.

Hypotonic

These rapidly replace fluids lost by sweating. Containing fluids, electrolytes and a very low level of carbohydrate, the main function of hypotonic drinks is hydration. They are suitable for strength and power athletes who do not need a boost of carbohydrate. Examples include Powerade Zero, Gatorade G2, and Amino Vital.

Isotonic

Isotonic drinks are the most popular choice for endurance athletes and team sports. They quickly replace fluids lost by sweating and supply a boost of carbohydrate. The carbohydrate source is typically supplied as glucose in a concentration of 6 to 8 percent. As glucose is the body's preferred source of energy, isotonic drinks are ideal for long workouts where a drop in blood glucose or muscle glycogen levels would result in decreased performance. Examples include Gatorade (original), Powerade (original) and Powerbar Endurance Sport drink.

Hypertonic

With a glucose concentration of 10 percent or more, these drinks are more food than fluid. They can be used to supplement daily carbohydrate intake, usually after exercise to top up muscle glycogen stores or during an ultradistance event where a greater level of fuelling required. If you do choose a hypertonic drink, consume plenty of plain water with it to hydrate. Examples include the Gatorade Performance Series and simple fruit juice.

Sports drinks can be expensive, so if you do decide they are the right choice for you, consider making your own with this quick and easy process. Simply add one pinch (1 gram) of salt to 1 litre of water and mix 100 millilitres, 200 millilitres or 400 millilitres of orange or lemon squash (made from concentrate) to create a hypotonic, isotonic or hypertonic drink, respectively. Mix well and keep the drink chilled. One advantage of a sports drink over plain water is the electrolytes it contains. However, correct food fuelling can also help balance electrolytes if you choose to rely on water alone for hydration.

WEIGHT-LOSS TIP If weight loss is your goal, stick to plain water rather than selecting a sports drink or juice, as the addition of carbohydrate before and during your workout only delays fat burning.

Your hydration levels pre workout can directly influence your performance, as even mild dehydration can reduce exercise intensity and duration. You can prevent the onset of dehydration during exercise by making sure you are well hydrated before starting. This does not mean glugging copious amounts of water immediately pre workout, which will simply leave you feeling uncomfortable and will dilute essential electrolytes (mainly sodium, which is important for muscle contractions). If you've ever experienced muscle cramps during exercise, you were quite likely lacking sodium.

The correct way to adequately hydrate pre workout is to drink water at regular intervals throughout the day, paying attention to the previously mentioned signs of dehydration. If you do need to compensate for any previously incurred fluid deficits, consume around 400 to 600 millilitres about 2 hours before your workout, and then continue to drink small amounts frequently up to the beginning of exercise and throughout it.

Fruit and vegetable juices are suitable in moderation during the day. Experiment with these as fluid options for immediately before your workout, perhaps diluting them with water to ensure you do not feel any sickness or other adverse effects during exercise. Good juice choices include tomato, apple, lemon and orange. Tomato juice in particular has added sodium, which may help address your electrolyte balance during endurance training and prevent cramps. Lemon juice increases the alkalinity of your body, which is especially beneficial as your body fluids become more acidic during exercise. This acidity has a number of negative consequences, including loss of calcium from bones if in a prolonged state of acidity.

SUPPLEMENTS

Supplements fall into different categories according to whether they claim to enhance performance (ergogenic), aid recovery or improve general health. A nutritious diet should provide all you need to perform well, recover fast and maintain good health. However, certain supplements may be appropriate for people at the top of their sporting game and for those whose nutrition is inadequate, which can be due to the deteriorated nutritional value of today's fruits, vegetables and grains from overfarming or from poor available choices (though we hope you will plan ahead and prepare foods ahead of time to avoid the latter).

This chapter cannot cover every supplement, since there are just so many on the market, but table 3.4 identifies our chosen selection of supplements, their benefits and advised dosage to help you to decide what could benefit your body.

SAMPLE MEAL PLANS FIT FOR PURPOSE

Select the daily menu suited to your activity. Whilst the menus in tables 3.2 and 3.3 both provide a good balance of fibrous carbohydrate, lean protein and healthy fat, our menu for strength athletes includes a larger protein component to further assist repair of natural muscle damage caused during strength training. The menu for endurance athletes leans towards a higher carbohydrate intake, as more of this macronutrient is required to sustain long bouts of aerobic exercise.

Table 3.2 Sample Daily Menu for a Strength Athlete

Breakfast	Scrambled eggs (1 or 2 whole, 3 whites) with spinach and berries
Lunch	Grilled turkey, green vegetable (broccoli, cabbage, asparagus) and avocado
Dinner	Baked chicken breast with roasted butternut squash, peppers, mushrooms, onion and a drizzle of olive oil

Snacks: 30 g raw nuts (walnuts, almonds, Brazil nuts) with apple, cottage cheese with ham or turkey slices, Dried beef snacks (beef jerky or biltong)	Fluids: 2 L or more

Table 3.3 Sample Daily Menu for an Endurance Athlete

Breakfast	Porridge oats with berries and seeds plus boiled egg
Lunch	Grilled turkey in wholemeal pitta bread with salad and avocado
Dinner	Salmon stir fry with green vegetable (broccoli, asparagus), peppers, onion, mushrooms and brown rice, plus a drizzle of olive oil

Snacks: Oatcakes × 2 with cottage cheese, dried apricots (25 g) and walnuts (25 g), Greek yoghurt with banana, honey and flaxseeds	Fluids: 2 L or more

Your individual daily calorie requirements and therefore quantities at each mealtime will depend on your body size, exercise duration and intensity, and weight loss or maintenance goals. Your fluid requirements also increase with activity. Don't forget to adapt these sample meal plans according to the timing of your workout and hence your pre- and postworkout needs. If your goal is weight loss, the strength athlete meal plan will have the best metabolic effect on fat burning and increasing lean tissue and help to achieve a calorie deficit without feeling hungry.

Table 3.4   Recommended Supplements for Women

Supplement	Benefits	Dosage
Omega-3s (fish oils)	Aids workout recovery, improves joint health, assists weight loss (in association with regular exercise), lowers high cortisol levels (your stress hormones produced during exercise) which encourage fat storage, reduces the risk of heart disease and is vitally important for healthy brain and cell function.	1,000 mg twice per day
Magnesium	Prevents sugar cravings, raises energy levels and assists workout recovery.	400 mg twice per day
Vitamin C	Speeds up recovery from the common cold, reduces cortisol and prevents urinary tract infections when taken in the form of ascorbic acid, as it helps acidify the urine and discourage bacterial growth.	500 mg twice per day
L-carnitine	Improves recovery from exercise and raises energy levels, enabling you to work harder and more frequently.	1,000 mg twice per day
L-glutamine	Facilitates the body's ability to burn fat for energy and helps overcome low energy, obesity and fatigue.	1,000 mg per day in powdered form, mixed into water
Glucosamine	Reduces joint pain associated with arthritis and injury; paired with the cartilage molecule chondroitin, it may help to slow osteoarthritis progression.	2,000 mg glucosamine daily or 1,500 mg glucosamine + 1,200 mg chondroitin daily
CoQ10	Involved in making the energy molecule adenosine triphosphate (ATP) needed to drive muscle contractions, helping you to exercise for longer. It's also an antioxidant, which scavenges free radicals and aids recovery from your workout.	100 mg twice per day
Iron	Builds bone and muscle and provides energy. Female athletes are at increased risk of iron deficiency because menstrual losses and deficiency can lead to long-term fatigue. However, supplementation may only be beneficial in women with actual iron-deficiency anaemia and not in nonanaemic athletes who have exhausted iron stores alone (prelatent iron deficiency), so identify which situation applies to you.	10–15 mg/day
Caffeine	Reduces fatigue and increases alertness, muscular power and endurance performance by enabling more fat to enter the bloodstream to be used as fuel, sparing the carbohydrate stores. Be aware of its diuretic effect and possible stomach upset, nervous jitters and headaches. Furthermore, its ergogenic effects will be greater if you abstain at certain times to prevent developing a tolerance.	3 mg per kg body weight (approx. equivalent of 1 Red Bull or 1 strong coffee for a 60 kg woman)

Supplement	Benefits	Dosage
Creatine	Increases muscle mass and strength and aids with short bursts of exercise such as sprinting and weightlifting when combined with appropriate training. It is particularly effective in performance of repeated bouts of exercise because it enhances recovery. However, it can cause bloating, especially in women, but products specifically designed for women reduce this effect.	3–5 mg/day

AT A GLANCE

- Eat 2 to 4 hours before exercise and include mostly low-GI carbohydrate, such as whole grains, combined with complete protein sources, such as eggs, to further slow the release of carbohydrate for energy. For an energy boost 10 minutes before exercise begins, choose an easily digested preworkout snack with a high-GI value, such as a banana or a sports drink.

- Consume 400 to 600 millilitres of water 2 hours before exercise if you have incurred any water deficit, and then continue to drink small amounts often leading up to and during your workout. Even mild dehydration can impair performance, so hydration is vitally important.

- Sports drinks are necessary only if you are exercising continuously for longer than 60 minutes or in extreme heat, if you have not adequately fuelled pre workout (especially during the morning) and if you focus on performance over weight loss. Otherwise, plain water is adequate. The three types of sports drinks are hypotonic, isotonic and hypertonic. Each contains varying levels of fluid, electrolytes and carbohydrate.

- Refuelling should begin during the 30-minute window after exercise with consumption of high-GI carbohydrate foods or sports drinks to instantly replace muscle glycogen. Add easily digested proteins, such as egg whites or whey protein drinks, to help resynthesis of muscle protein, which is naturally broken down during strenuous exercise.

- Refuelling should continue with a whole-food meal 2 to 4 hours post workout and throughout the rest of the day with nutrition that suits your needs as an endurance or strength-based athlete. Combine low-GI carbohydrate with lean protein sources and good fats rich in omega-3 in each meal.

- Body-weight loss after exercise is a good indicator of dehydration, and it can be used to determine fluid consumption. A 1-kilogram loss is equal to 1 litre of water. Consume 150 percent of your loss during the

(continued)

(continued)

hours that follow exercise to be sure of rehydration. Replace electrolytes with sports drinks or salty snacks.

- Your requirement for supplements depends on the type and intensity of your workout as well as the quality of your diet. Supplements can aid performance (ergogenic), such as caffeine and creatine; help recovery, such as L-carnitine and magnesium; or simply improve general health, such as omega-3 fish oils. Choose supplements that suit your requirements, but do not use them as a substitute for good nutrition.

Warming Up and Cooling Down

4

A good warm-up and cool-down are undoubtedly an essential part of any workout, and we all know we should include them. Why, then, do so many of us take shortcuts by performing a token swing of our arms and some toe touches or even bypassing any attempt altogether? The answer is usually time restraints or a lack of understanding of what to do. When time is limited, we are keen to get on with our workout and get back to work, home or study. Warming up and cooling down take additional time, effort and understanding. But before you skip onto the next chapter, consider this: If you are serious about your workout or sport, then time spent on warming up and cooling down effectively is time well spent, as both have the following proven benefits:

- Enhance performance
- Prevent injury
- Increase total calorie burn to help weight loss or weight management
- Aid recovery
- Address and correct any muscular imbalances

So now that we've established that this is a must-do part of any successful training programme, let us guide you through the different stages of your warm-up and cool-down, explain the benefits of each and provide specific examples for you to try. Your warm-up and cool-down involve different stages, and various methods are available for each. We will explore the incorporation of cardiorespiratory exercises, joint mobilisation, various stretching techniques and movement drills, including pre-activation and even mental-preparation techniques for warm-up and further recovery aids for the cool-down. We will also look at the recent trend for utilising vibration training to further enhance your preparation, recovery and conditioning.

WARM-UP

The main purpose of any warm-up is to improve your performance in the workout, sport or competitive event to follow, and several benefits of warming up help you to do just that.

Increased Heart Rate

Beginning exercise at a workable rate increases blood flow around your body, delivering oxygen and vital energy components to your muscles.

Increased Muscle Temperature

Temperature increases in the muscles being warmed up, allowing them to contract more forcefully and relax more quickly, allowing for greater speed and strength. Furthermore, a warm muscle is more pliable and less likely to be overstretched and injured. Think of your muscles as elastic bands—a warm band is more springy and reactive than a cold band, which is more likely to snap when under tension!

Increased Blood Temperature

As blood travels through the active muscles, its temperature rises and the binding of oxygen to haemoglobin weakens so oxygen is more readily available to working muscles. This has the potential to improve your endurance.

Increased Range of Motion (ROM)

A good workout increases the range of motion and mobility of a joint, allowing more efficient movement and helping to prevent injury.

Increased Muscle Activation

Performing pre-activation exercises as part of your warm-up puts your muscles in a state of readiness, which stimulates nerves, speeds up neural transmission and readies muscles to respond faster and more efficiently. This is most beneficial ahead of a workout relying on speed and power.

Hormonal Stimulation

During the warm-up, your body increases its production of the different hormones responsible for regulating energy production. This balance of hormones makes more carbohydrates and fatty acids available for energy production.

Blood Vessel Dilation

This occurs in response to your rise in body temperature and reduces both the resistance to blood flow and the stress on your heart.

Mental Preparation

The warm-up process is great for getting into the zone with mind techniques, such as mental rehearsal and imagery, and for giving you the confidence that you are physically ready to perform or train at your best.

Now that you're happy with why it's important to warm up before exercise, let's look at how to do it. The four stages of a warm-up typically include the following:

1. *Light cardiorespiratory exercise*: 5–10 minutes
2. *Dynamic stretching exercises*: 5–10 minutes
3. *Exercise drills*: 5–10 minutes
4. *Mental preparation*: 5–10 minutes

The time, relevance and emphasis you place on each part of the warm-up very much depend on the nature and intensity of the activity or event to follow. The warm-up can be as short as 10 minutes prior to a cardio-respiratory gym session where you include stages 1 and 2 only or as long as 40 minutes or more prior to a competition where all four stages are completed. We will now look into the details of each stage and provide examples for each one.

Stage 1: Light Cardiorespiratory Exercise

This first stage of the warm-up is 5 to 10 minutes of light cardio, which increases heart rate and the temperature of the body, blood and muscles as described previously. You choose the mode of exercise, which should be general in nature at this stage. Examples include jogging, cycling, cross-trainer, rowing or skipping. At this stage, runners can jog, but play around by adding skips forwards, sideways and backwards to warm and activate your muscles from all angles. You can even swing your arms as you do so to further raise your heart rate and incorporate your upper body. If you are trying to reduce impact-based activity because of knee or back injuries, then a cycle or cross-trainer may be a better option for you. Again, incorporate movements with your upper body and vary the tempo as your muscles start to warm up.

During this stage, the intensity should be light. As such, you should be able to hold a conversation without feeling uncomfortable or out of breath. We like to use a rating of perceived exertion (RPE) scale to guide your effort level during cardiorespiratory warm-ups. Use the following 10-point scale for reference and aim for a rating between 3 and 4 as a rough guide.

Figure 4.1   Rating of Perceived Exertion (RPE) Scale

RPE number	Breathing rate/ability to talk	Exertion
1	Resting	Very slight
2	Talking is easy	Slight
3	Talking is easy	Moderate
4	You can talk but with more effort	Somewhat hard
5	You can talk but with more effort	Hard
6	Breathing is challenged/don't want to talk	Hard
7	Breathing is challenged/don't want to talk	Very hard
8	Panting hard/conversation is difficult	Very hard
9	Panting hard/conversation is difficult	Very, very hard
10	Cannot sustain this intensity for too long	Maximal

Reprinted, by permission, from K. Austin and B. Seebohar, 2011, *Performance nutrition: Applying the science of nutrient timing* (Champaign, IL: Human Kinetics), 30.

Stage 2: Dynamic Stretching Exercises

Now that you have warmed your muscles, the second stage of the warm-up involves 5 to 10 minutes of dynamic stretching. This stage of the warm-up is about lengthening your muscles to the degree that you will use them in your subsequent activity or event, increasing the range of motion around the joint and addressing any muscle imbalances. Stretching beyond the desired range for your activity provides no benefit as you are not likely to have the strength at the extreme ranges. You will suffer reduced performance or, worse still, strained muscles.

You can choose from a number of stretching techniques, including static, dynamic, passive and active stretches and their variations. We have included a review of each type of stretching in the following section. Familiarise yourself with the terms and techniques before reading our discussion of why dynamic stretches are most suitable at this stage.

STRETCHING TERMS AND TECHNIQUES

Several stretching terms and techniques exist, and each is performed in a different way and at a different time depending on your desired outcome.

Static Stretching

A static stretch (e.g., seated straight-leg toe touch) is held in a fixed position (challenging but comfortable) for a set period of time (usually up to 30 seconds). It is the most commonly used stretch for safely improving overall flexibility.

Dynamic Stretching

A dynamic stretch (e.g., forward and backward alternating leg swings) is performed by repeatedly moving through a challenging but comfortable range of motion for a set number of repetitions (e.g., 10 to 12). It is ideal for improving functional range of motion and mobility for sports and daily activities. The controlled, smooth and deliberate movement should not be confused with *ballistic stretching* (remember bouncing toe touches from your school physical education lessons), which is uncontrolled and jerky, and is likely to lead to injury.

Passive Stretching

A passive stretch (e.g., stretching the hamstring while lying down, hooking a band around your foot, and using the held end to pull your leg towards your body) is achieved using some external assistance such as your body weight, a strap or resistance band, gravity, stretching device or even another person. You relax the muscle to be stretched whilst the external force holds you in place. This technique can be used for both static and dynamic stretches. It is a relatively easy and relaxed way to stretch, provided the external force being used doesn't push you into too much discomfort or beyond your desired range of motion.

Active Stretching

An active stretch (e.g., kneeling hip and quad stretch, whereby you contract your gluteal muscle on the side being stretched to assist and enhance the stretch) is achieved by actively contracting the opposing muscle to the one you are stretching whilst the stretched muscle is relaxed. Although no external assistance is necessary here, active stretching can be challenging due to the muscular strength required to generate the stretch. However, as you are controlling the stretch force internally (with your own force), the risk of overstretching is very low compared to those using external assistance. This technique can be used for both static and dynamic stretches.

(continued)

(continued)

Proprioceptive Neuromuscular Facilitation (PNF) Stretching

PNF stretching (e.g., a lying-down hamstring stretch whereby a person pushes your leg towards you whilst you resist by pushing back against them) is a combination of the four preceding techniques. It is generally thought to be one of the most effective forms of stretching for flexibility and generating a fast muscle relaxation response. To perform this technique, apply force using the muscle being stretched against an external source (usually a partner) whilst they resist and push back for 5 to 10 seconds. As your muscle gradually lengthens, you progress the stretch to a greater range, relaxing between each effort and repeating the contraction.

It has recently become clear that static stretching (the technique most commonly used to stretch) is not beneficial before exercise. Studies suggest, alarmingly, that people who perform these stretches before physical activity may even have a higher rate of injury than those who don't! Static stretches may also reduce the ability of the muscles to produce power and force, which may be necessary for those of you about to perform a weight training or circuit training session and for those participating in sports such as tennis, netball and athletics. This is because in the moments immediately following a static stretch, the soft tissue is not as responsive as it might have been before the stretch. It has in effect lost its excitability and reactiveness. Therefore, static stretching can diminish performance.

We expect many of you reading this book have come to rely on static stretches as a familiar precursor to exercise. We have also done the same at various stages of our athletic careers. You may therefore feel reluctant and even vulnerable leaving these out altogether. But before you sadly abandon static stretching, we want to put it in context and reassure you that it still has its place, but that place is post exercise, when the muscles are fully warm and no longer required to produce power, or as a primary focus session such as some forms of Pilates and yoga. Improvements only come with adaptation, so try changing when you use static stretches and note changes in performance and recovery.

Now we've established that static stretching is not ideal during the warm-up stage, we will turn our attention back to our prescription of dynamic stretching exercises. As part of the overall warm-up, dynamic stretches will in fact improve performance and reduce the risk of injury as they gradually and progressively stimulate and replicate the more stressful activity to follow. Dynamic stretches, even if not sports-specific at this stage, enhance total body range of motion and further increase tissue temperature.

The following stretches incorporate multiple muscle groups. They are suitable both before an all-over body gym workout and before sporting activity. These stretches are all dynamic and suitable for intermediate to advanced exercisers. The main muscles targeted and the purpose of the stretch are indicated for each one. Each stretch repetition should take 1 to 3 seconds. Repeat the movement continuously in a controlled and smooth manner 10 to 12 times. For each stretch, exhale as you move into the stretch position and inhale each time you release the stretch. For those dynamic stretches that are more continuous, aim for a general controlled state of breathing throughout that matches the rhythm of the movement. These stretches are examples, and we advise you pick and choose those that suit your activity needs and address areas in which you particularly lack flexibility.

DYNAMIC SIDE-TO-SIDE LUNGE WITH ARM REACH

Exercise Focus

Adductors, latissimus dorsi and trunk lateral flexors

How To

Stand with your feet wide apart and your toes at 45 degrees. Bend one knee and lunge to that side, reaching the opposite arm over your head simultaneously and keeping the opposite leg straight (see figure 4.2*a*). Use your free arm to support your body weight on the thigh if needed. Then, reach and lunge immediately to the other side (see figure 4.2*b*). Continue to alternate lunging and reaching from left to right.

Contract the gluteal muscle on the side opposite to the one being stretched to control lunging depth and avoid leaning forward or back.

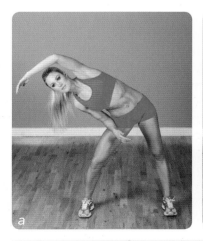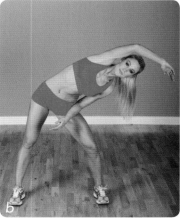

Figure 4.2   Dynamic side-to-side lunge with arm reach.

QIGONG TOE TOUCH

Exercise Focus

Hamstrings, gastrocnemius and erector spinae

How To

Stand with your feet together and slide your hands down your legs, bending your knees (see figure 4.3a). Place your hands directly over your toes, keeping the fingers aligned with the toes. Raise your hips up and roll slightly back on your heels to straighten your legs (see figure 4.3b). Drop down again, rolling forward towards the balls of your feet. Repeat.

*A*void fully and forcefully locking your knees on the extension.

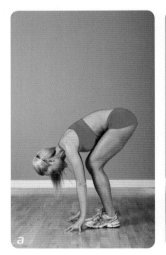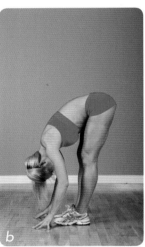

Figure 4.3   Qigong toe touch.

FORWARD TO BACKWARD LEG SWINGS

Exercise Focus

Hip flexors, quadriceps, glutes and hamstrings

Equipment

Wall or fixed object

How To

Stand up straight with your feet together and your side to a wall, tree or other fixed object. Hold on to the object with your nearest arm for support. With a swinging motion, straighten the leg farther away from the wall and extend it behind you (see figure 4.4a). Then, immediately swinging it back in front of your body (see figure 4.4b). Perform continuously, swinging the leg from back to front with a pendulum movement whilst keeping your anchor leg strong but slightly flexed. Repeat on the other side.

Work to avoid outward hip rotation during the backward phase by keeping your hips forward throughout the movement.

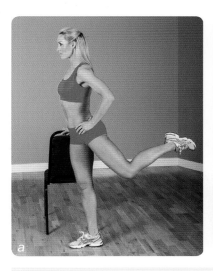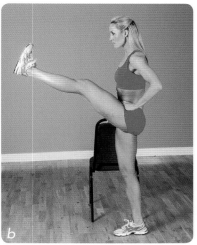

Figure 4.4   Forward to backward leg swings.

LATERAL LEG SWINGS

Exercise Focus

Adductors, abductors, glutes and hip rotators

Equipment

Wall or fixed object

How To

Stand up straight with your feet together, face a wall, tree or other fixed object, and support yourself with both hands. Lift one leg, bending it 90 degrees at the knee, and swing it across your body (see figure 4.5a). Then, immediately swing it back in the opposite direction and out to the side of your body (see figure 4.5b). Perform continuously, swinging the leg from one side to the other. To progress this stretch, allow the swinging leg to extend at the knee as it moves out to the side at the point where the foot is farthest away from the body. Rise up on the ball of the foot of the supporting leg to allow the swinging leg to move more freely without contacting the ground.

> **K**eep your hips facing forward throughout the movement.

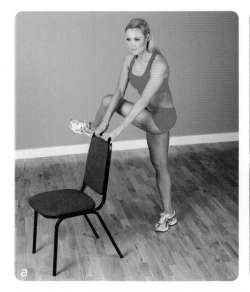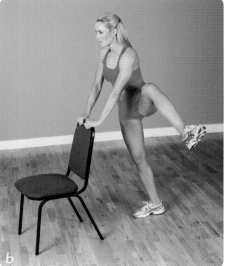

Figure 4.5   Lateral leg swings.

DYNAMIC CALF STRETCH

Exercise Focus

Calves

Equipment

Wall or fixed object

How To

With your feet together, lean your body forwards and press your hands against a wall, tree or other fixed object for support. Keeping your body straight, walk your feet backwards to the farthest point where you can keep your heels on the ground while still touching the support-ing object. Keeping both feet in contact with the ground, raise one heel and push your weight into the heel still touching the ground (see figure 4.6a). Switch legs (see figure 4.6b). Alternate pushing and lifting your feet, shifting your weight from one side to the other.

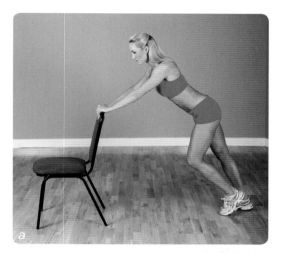

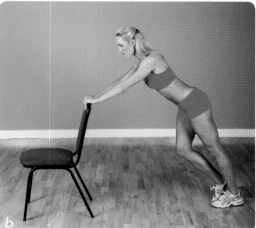

Figure 4.6   Dynamic calf stretch.

DYNAMIC ROLL AND REACH

Exercise Focus

Erector spinae, glutes and hamstrings

How To

Sit on the floor with your knees bent and your hands holding onto your shins, and pull your thighs close to your chest (see figure 4.7*a*). Tuck your chin to your chest and roll backwards until your shoulder blades touch the floor (see figure 4.7*b*). Immediately roll back into a seated position, extending your legs in front of your body and reaching your arms forwards to touch your toes (see figure 4.7*c*). Return to the start position and repeat, working to move your chest progressively closer to your thighs with each leg extension.

Keep your neck and shoulders relaxed.

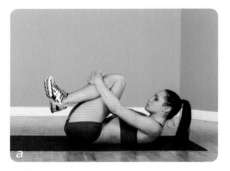

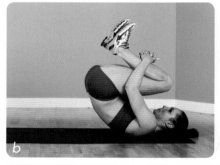

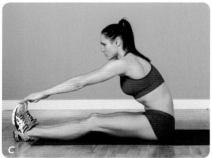

Figure 4.7   Dynamic roll and reach.

ARM SWINGS ACROSS CHEST

Exercise Focus

Deltoids and pectorals

How To

Stand with your feet shoulder-width apart and arms outstretched to either side of your body. With a fluid movement, swing both arms across your chest, crossing one over the other during the movement (see figure 4.8*a*). Then immediately swing them back and behind your body, lifting your chest as you go (see figure 4.8*b*). Perform continuously, increasing your range with each repetition.

Avoid rounding your spine.

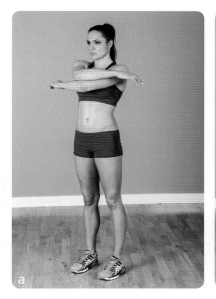 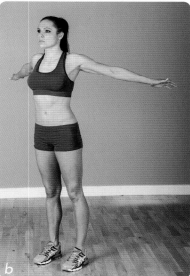

Figure 4.8   Arm swings across chest.

DYNAMIC STANDING FIGURE-FOUR STRETCH

Exercise Focus

Glutes and piriformis

Equipment

Wall or fixed object

How To

Stand with your feet slightly apart and hold a fixed object in front of you for support. Place one foot across the thigh of your opposite leg in a figure-four position (see figure 4.9*a*) and squat down to a 90-degree knee bend (see figure 4.9*b*). Stand up and move out of the squat position, keeping your foot on your thigh. Repeat the down and up movement. The deeper you sit into the stretch, the greater the stretch you will achieve. Repeat with the other leg.

Keep your back flat and your head facing forwards.

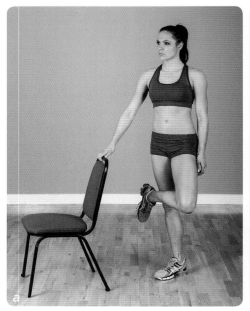 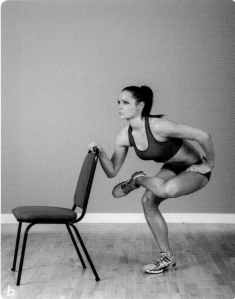

Figure 4.9   Dynamic standing figure-four stretch.

LYING SPINAL ROTATIONS

Exercise Focus

Erector spinae, glutes and pectorals

How To

Lie on your back with your knees bent and arms extended to each side of your body. Rotate your hips and knees, lowering them to the floor on one side of your body, and move your head and neck in the op-posite direction (see figure 4.10*a*). Then immediately lift and move your knees up and across to the other side of your body, again moving your head and neck in the op-posite direction (see figure 4.10*b*). Repeat continuously.

Keep both shoulders pressed to the ground as you move from side to side.

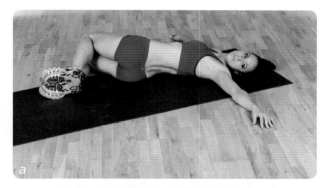

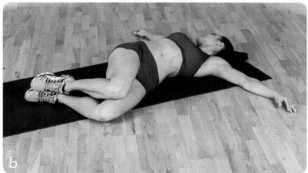

Figure 4.10   Lying spinal rotations.

DYNAMIC KNEELING LATISSIMUS STRETCH

Exercise Focus

Latissimus dorsi

Equipment

Swiss ball

How To

Kneel on the floor and place your forearms on a Swiss ball about half a metre in front of you (see figure 4.11a). Bend at the hips and push your shoulders towards the floor, allowing the ball to roll away from you until you feel an optimum stretch down both sides of your body (see figure 4.11b). Lift your hips back to the start position and repeat continuously.

> **A**pply more force into the ball on the downward phase of the movement for a greater stretch.

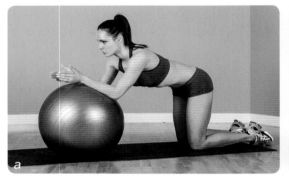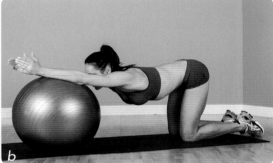

Figure 4.11   Dynamic kneeling latissimus stretch on a ball.

Try out all of the preceding dynamic stretching exercises to discover which best suit your activities and particular flexibility and mobility needs. Your stretching requirements will vary depending on your level of conditioning, existing flexibility and joint mobility, the surrounding temperature, previous injury considerations and the demands and nature of the workout to follow. If you are about to perform a cardiorespiratory, steady-state elliptical workout, for example, you would perform fewer stretches and choose those of a more general nature than if you were preparing to take part in sport. Further, the sport to be performed, whether it involves predominantly upper or lower body exercises, repetitive movements or power efforts, multidirectional movements and rotations or linear movements, will also dictate the stretches you choose. Become familiar with your own requirements and choose your warm-up stretches accordingly.

Stage 3: Exercise Drills

This stage of the warm-up is most appropriate for those preparing for sport, for any exercise involving load and for power-based exercises. These may include running, tennis, weightlifting and sprinting. The purpose of stage 3 is to spend 5 to 10 minutes preparing yourself for action by moving your now warmed and mobilised muscles and joints through patterns that imitate those you are about to perform during your session. If you were to go straight into a tennis match after a cardiorespiratory warm-up and some dynamic stretching, you would not have fully activated the muscles and neural pathways necessary for efficient movement patterns in tennis. You will often see a track athlete doing various skips, high knees and extended strides before a full-out sprint. Likewise, a weightlifter will begin her session with light lifts (perhaps at 50 to 60 percent of her max) before increasing the load.

Exercise drills essentially preactivate the muscles needed for your sport or activity so that they contract faster, more explosively and with better efficiency. As such, these drills should not create fatigue or excess stress, and you should feel recovered prior to each effort. They also provide you with the confidence that your body is ready to perform optimally and without restriction and they can help to increase the level of conditioning of your muscles.

Suitable drills exist for both the lower and upper body and for different sports. We will explore these now and provide examples for you to try and to incorporate into your own warm-up when required. The following drills are general in nature and as such are suitable before an all-over body workout or sporting activity. Perform each drill over 20 to 30 metres. Perform 1 to 3 sets of the drills (building this number of sets at 2-week intervals). To recover, walk back or jog gently between drills; rest for 5 minutes between sets.

HEEL-TO-TOE WALKING KNEE DRIVE

Drill Focus

Calves

How To

Plant the heel of one foot out in front of you and leverage your weight over this leg whilst keeping the leg straight (see figure 4.12a). Next, drive your weight forward, rising up onto the ball of the planted foot, and bringing your other leg up to knee drive position (see figure 4.12b). Perform continuously from one foot to the other.

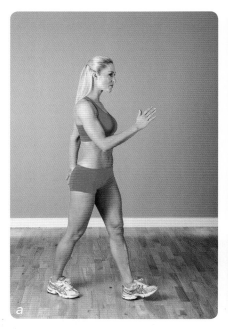 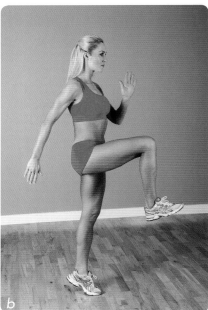

Figure 4.12   Heel-to-toe walking knee drive.

BUM KICKS

Drill Focus

Hamstrings and calves

How To

Standing tall on the balls of your feet, kick your feet backwards one at a time, flicking your heel to touch the corresponding cheek of your bottom (see figure 4.13) and moving forwards as you alternate feet. Drive your arms in a running motion.

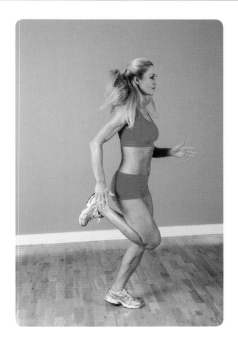

Figure 4.13 Bum kicks.

HIGH-KNEE SKIPS

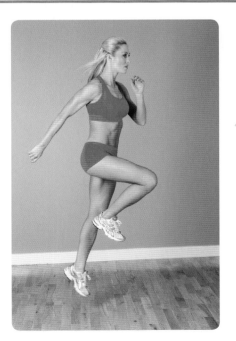

Drill Focus

Calves, quadriceps and glutes

How To

Perform a standard skipping motion, driving off the back leg and raising the opposite knee up and forwards (see figure 4.14). Land with soft knees and then drive off with the opposite leg. Continue the process, alternating legs. Remember to drive up the arm opposite to the lifting leg.

Figure 4.14 High-knee skips.

SIDE HEEL TAP SKIPS

Drill Focus

Calves, adductors, quadriceps, glutes and abductors

How To

Stand sideways and with the feet together. Step one leg out to the side and plant it to the ground to lead the movement (see figure 4.15a). Next, push off and up from this lead leg, bringing the trail leg up to tap heels together at your highest point in the air (see figure 4.15b). Land with the weight on the trail leg and step onto the lead leg again to repeat the movement (see figure 4.15c). Repeat leading with the opposite leg.

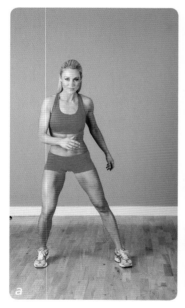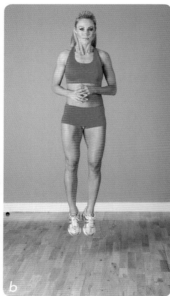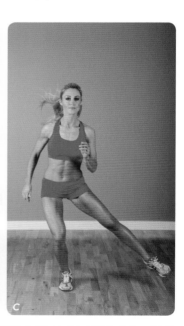

Figure 4.15   Side heel tap skips.

BACKWARD LUNGES

Drill Focus

Quadriceps, calves and glutes

How To

Start with the feet together, then lift one foot (see figure 4.16*a*) and place it behind you into a lunge, keeping your hips and chest facing forward (see figure 4.16*b*). Push off the front foot and place it behind you in a lunge position on the opposite side. Continue alternating legs for reverse lunges, working your arms in conjunction with your legs for balance and co-ordination.

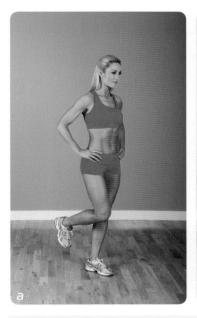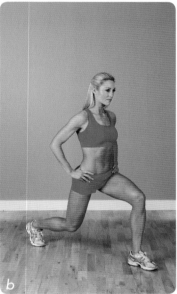

Figure 4.16   Backward lunge.

Stage 4: Mental Preparation

There's just one more thing to do before you begin your workout or competition, and that is to train your brain. We're talking about being as mentally prepared as you are physically. Mental preparation is frequently overlooked, yet it can make the difference between an average session or race and a spectacular one. Some benefits of mental preparation include the following:

- Creating the perfect pre-event state—arousal, relaxation, concentration and energy
- Improving technical skills (even when injured and unable to train physically)
- Counteracting negative images and mistakes
- Developing game tactics
- Gaining confidence in your abilities

The purpose of mental preparation is to create the state required to train or perform at your best. This ideal state will vary from person to person and from one activity to another. The process is sometimes referred to as 'getting into the zone'. A boxer, for example, will typically want to create a state of maximum arousal and controlled aggression, whilst a tae kwon do athlete and high jumper may require a calm, clear head. Remember, mental preparation is not just reserved for competition. Mentally preparing for any workout, whether it is a long cycle ride or a circuit training session, will mean you push harder, work more efficiently and ultimately achieve greater results and satisfaction. There's nothing more frustrating than watching someone going through the motions of a training session without fully maximising her efforts. Training time is your time and your chance to be the best you can be.

We want to focus on three mental preparation practices here: imagery, self-talk and physical movement. Try them and discover which works best for you. You may find you are already doing some of these without even realising it!

Imagery

Imagery, sometimes referred to as visualisation, uses the power of your imagination. This is the process of mentally mimicking real physical rehearsal. It works by programming your muscles to react in the way that you want, as simply thinking about doing an action creates neural patterns in your brain that induce micro muscle movements that mimic what will actually happen when you perform that action.

Imagery uses all of your senses (sight, sound, touch, taste and smell). The clearer and more controllable your mental images are, the more effective your mental preparation will be. We all have a preferred way of thinking and will favour drawing on certain representative systems, or senses, more than others. We might practice imagery in two distinctly different ways:

- *Association*—Picture the action or event, as seen from your own eyes and body. Mental rehearsal must be associated to be effective. Your muscles respond to your images only when you imagine them in terms of your own body.
- *Dissociation*—Watch yourself from outside your body, as though you're viewing yourself in a picture or movie. This is a good learning practice that is useful for setting up mental rehearsal.

With this understanding, you can mentally prepare using the following sequence:

1. *Imagine your race or workout environment.* If this is a gym, running track or games field, for example, then picture any equipment, including its positioning, colours, and dimensions, as well as any people who may be present, whether competitors or friends and family.

2. *Visualise your technique or skill using dissociation.* Whether you need to shoot a goal in netball or complete a 5,000-metre rowing time trial in your gym, watch yourself going through the different movement patterns required and create a picture of fluidity and ease between the movements.

3. *Mentally rehearse with associated imagery.* Now do the exercise, visualising from inside your body. Go through the movement pattern in your mind, almost feeling your body and relevant muscles in action. Do this several times until you feel you've accomplished a great execution of the movement or activity.

Now set up and rehearse these components, which are important for the effective use of imagery for any event or practice:

- *Set your goal*—Your goal may be running 10K on the treadmill or executing the perfect tennis game where you win in 2 sets. Whatever it is, make sure you've made it clear. Refer back to Chapter 1: Training Essentials, for advice on setting your goals.

- *Focus on the process, not the end result*—This means breaking down your goal into manageable stages and skills to help you physically and mentally on your way to achieving it. For an open water swim, the processes may include changing the length of your stroke to overcome the large waves, adjusting to the temperature of the water and executing the movement patterns of your chosen stroke. The result will then come naturally.

- *Be specific at each stage*—Understand and have a clear picture of every stage of your event or practice. This may include how much time you have to warm up, how many competitors you will face, how you will execute the first move and so forth. Don't leave anything to chance, as you will likely feel panicked and underprepared during the performance. Without a clear picture of every stage, your visualisation technique will be compromised.

- *Visualise perfection*—As you begin to visualise your event or practice, imagine everything as you want it to be. Your preparation process, execution and result are perfect.

- *Use all of your senses*—Hear the sounds, breathe the fresh air and feel your sense of balance. The more senses you use, the more memorable the experience will be.

- *Relax*—Find a place where you can visualise without distraction, as relaxation enhances the effects.

- *Practice*—Perfect practice makes perfect performance. Imagery is a skill like any other, so the more perfect practice you do, the more skilled you will become and the better your results will be. No set rule exists as to when to perform visualisation, but a good guide is to aim to do a 10-minute imagery session 2 or 3 times per week, incorporating parts of this into your warm-up.

Self-Talk

Self-talk reflects the link between your thoughts and performance. This strategy uses self-addressed cues (words or short phrases) to trigger appropriate responses and actions that improve performance. It is helpful for both focusing your attention and psyching up.

Different types of self-talk have been identified by researchers. You can call on them as the situation requires and to suit your particular needs.

- *Instructional self-talk*—This instruction is technical and is most suitable for tasks involving fine skills. For example, a hurdler may say 'Keep your elbow tucked in' whilst negotiating the barriers and a novice tennis player would repeat 'Keep your eye on the ball at all times.'

- *Motivational self-talk*—This is most suitable prior to tasks involving strength or endurance, and is used for boosting confidence and for psyching up. You may have heard athletes shouting 'Give it all you've got', 'Destroy the field', or 'Eat up the track!'

It is often said that self-talk has a greater effect on fine skills (putting a ball) than gross skills (running or swimming), as it mainly improves concentration, but this really depends on you as an individual and what you respond best to.

Self-talk is also believed to be most effective at the early stages of learning a sport or new movement pattern because learning takes place faster and more easily at these stages. Nonetheless it can be a valuable tool for both novices and experienced athletes because as you prepare your scripts and practice regularly, you will enhance your self-belief and performance.

Physical Movement

This technique does not refer to the physical warm-up you perform for cardiorespiratory exercise, stretching and drills, but rather the physical presence, actions or demeanour that you display prior to a race, maximal lift or effort to ready yourself for action. For example, if you compare video of the final race preparations of sprinter Usain Bolt to those of Michael Johnson before stepping into the starting blocks, you will see two very different approaches. Whilst Bolt made jokes and pulled his signature moves to the crowd, Johnson would simply stand very calm and still. It is clear that whilst Bolt required energy and excitement to feel mentally prepared, Johnson sought inner focus, blocking out everything around him. So the final physical movements you display, either with the purpose of helping yourself get into state or disturbing that of your competitors, has to be specific to you and what comes naturally.

What you are visualising (imagery), saying (self-talk) or doing (physical movement) needs to be congruent with what you believe and what you want. There is no point shouting 'I'm the best' if inside you're feeling embarrassed for doing so and totally insecure. Congruence, or making sure your delivery matches your meaning, will enable you to truly maximise the potential of mental preparation.

COOL-DOWN

The purpose of a cool-down is to gradually return your body to its resting state and to reduce the chances of muscle soreness in the days that follow. An effective cool-down has the following benefits:

- *Removes toxins*—Keeping your blood flowing post exercise with light cardiorespiratory exercise, rather than abruptly stopping movement, increases lymphatic flow that will remove the waste products that build up during exercise, namely lactic acid.

- *Reduces the potential for delayed-onset muscle soreness (DOMS)*—The requirement here is to reduce the inflammation to nerve endings and deliver nutrients to your muscles for repair and recovery. A cool-down can potentially do this by increasing blood flow and removing toxins. See the sidebar for more detail on DOMS.

- *Prevents chances of dizziness or fainting*—These unpleasant effects are caused by the pooling of venous blood if you stop exercising abruptly.

- *Reduces adrenaline levels in the blood*—This acts to reduce the stress levels of your body, as adrenaline and cortisol, produced during exercise, are stress hormones.

- *Lowers heart rate to resting level*—This helps return all your bodily functions—breathing, hormones and body temperature—to normal.

UNDERSTANDING DELAYED-ONSET MUSCLE SORENESS (DOMS)

DOMS is an unpleasant feeling that often lasts a couple of days after any exercise where you have worked your muscles harder or in a different way to what you are familiar with. Here's a little more information to understand the process and how to minimise its effects:

- DOMS describes the experience of muscle soreness, pain or stiffness that occurs 24 to 48 hours after exercise.
- It is most likely to be experienced when you begin a new exercise programme, change your exercise routine or significantly increase the duration or intensity of your workout.
- DOMS is a normal response to extreme exertion and is part of an adaptation process that leads to greater endurance and strength as muscles recover and build.
- It is caused by microscopic tearing of the muscle fibres. The extent of tearing, and soreness, depends on the intensity and type of the exercise done.
- Eccentric muscle contractions, movements that cause the muscle to forcefully contract as it lengthens, seem to cause the most soreness, as they increase intracellular pressure that irritates the nerve endings, causing swelling and local pain. Examples of eccentric contractions include running downhill and slowly lowering a weight under tension.
- DOMS can be reduced by performing a good warm-up and cool-down and using additional recovery methods, all described in this chapter.

The three main stages of a cool-down include the following:

1. *Light cardiorespiratory exercise*: 5 to 10 minutes
2. *Static stretches*: 5 to 10 minutes
3. *Recovery methods*: time depends on technique

As stated for the warm-up, the time and emphasis you place on your cool-down will depend on the workout performed, with more intense and enduring workouts necessitating a more substantial cool-down. We will address these three stages now, providing examples for you to try.

Stage 1: Light Cardiorespiratory Exercise

This first stage of your cool-down will prevent your blood from pooling, which leads to dizziness and fainting, and will reduce your body temperature, heart rate and breathing rate gradually. Consequently, you should gradually decrease the intensity of this cardio exercise, slowly reducing your pace and range of motion.

To cool down the right muscles, choose a modality that mimics the one you have been using during your workout. However, this is a personal choice. You may wish to use a nonimpact modality if you have been running and are feeling some tenderness or stress from impact. The most commonly used cardio cool-down modalities are jogging, walking, cycling and gliding on a cross-trainer. Whichever modality you choose, aim to reduce the resistance, range and pace. If you are jogging, then transition to a brisk walk after a few minutes and lower your arms to perform a simple swinging motion to help reduce your heart rate before finally stopping.

Stage 2: Static Stretching

We have already established that static stretching is most effective when performed as part of your cool-down, as it helps the muscles to relax, realigns muscle fibres and re-establishes their normal range of motion. Your muscles will already be warm and pliable from your previous activity and cardiorespiratory cool-down, so you can now focus on a deeper and more beneficial stretch to all your major muscles.

Perform a total-body stretch routine at this stage, playing particular attention to the specific muscles you have used during your exercise or sport. Hold each stretch for 10 seconds (30 seconds if done as part of a stand-alone stretching session), remembering to stretch both sides of your body. Begin by simply holding your stretch position at the level whereby you feel slight discomfort but not pain. As this level of discomfort eases, push slightly further into the stretch. Try the contract–relax method, or PNF method described earlier in this chapter, to further enhance and progress your stretch. Exhale as you move into the stretch position and inhale each time you release the stretch.

Try our pick of the best static stretches and incorporate into your cool down routine. The main muscles targeted are indicated for each stretch.

SEATED STRADDLE

Exercise Focus

Adductors and latissimus dorsi

How To

Sit on the floor with your legs straight. Position them as wide apart as possible whilst still keeping your chest upright. With your back flat, arms outstretched and head neutral, lower your chest between your legs (see figure 4.17).

Keep your knees slightly bent for comfort and ease gently into the stretch.

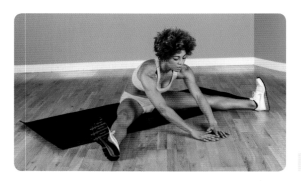

Figure 4.17   Seated straddle.

COBRA

Exercise Focus

Abdominals

How To

Lie on your belly with your hands just outside the tops of your shoulders (see figure 4.18a). Raise your upper body, pushing up with your hands and keeping your hips pressed into the floor (see figure 4.18b).

Relax your back muscles.

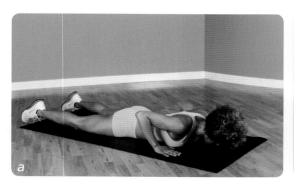
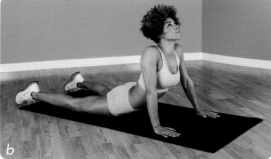

Figure 4.18   Cobra.

KNEELING LUNGE WITH REACH

Exercise Focus

Hip flexors, latissimus dorsi and obliques

How To

Assume a lunge position and drop your back knee to lightly rest on the floor. Move your hips forwards, keeping them square to the front. To increase the stretch further, reach the arm on the side you are stretching over your head and bend your trunk to that same side (see figure 4.19).

To maximise the hip flexor stretch, draw your navel in towards your spine and tuck your tailbone under to flatten your lower back before moving into position.

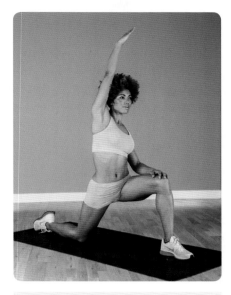

Figure 4.19   Kneeling lunge with reach.

90–90 HIP STRETCH

Exercise Focus

Glutes, piriformis and erector spinae

How To

Sit on the floor with both your legs bent to 90 degrees, maintaining the angle with the position of your groin. Place your hands on the ground on either side of your hips (see figure 4.20*a*). Keeping your back flat, lower your chest over your front leg until you feel a comfortable stretch in your outer thigh and hip (see figure 4.20*b*). You can use your hand to press your front knee and ankle firmly into the ground for the last few seconds of the stretch. Try leaning across over your ankle to change the angle of the stretch and to target a different part of your gluteal muscles (see figure 4.20*c*). If you are lacking in hip flexibility, you can adjust the angle of your front knee to 45 degrees.

As you lean forwards into the stretch, do so with a flat back, avoiding an arched and strained reaching position.

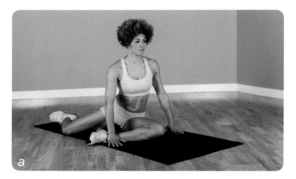

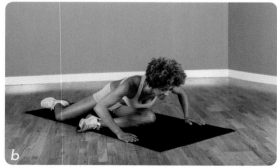
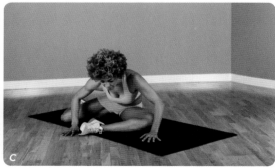

Figure 4.20   90–90 hip stretch.

DOWNWARD FACING DOG

Exercise Focus

Calves, hamstrings, abdominals and pectorals

How To

Stand with your feet together, then place both hands flat on the floor in front of you and walk them out to a distance whereby your heels remain on the floor. Slowly push your chest downwards and your hips backwards to transfer your weight through your

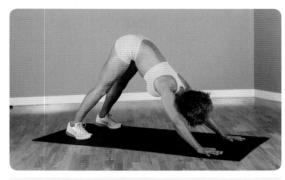

Figure 4.21   Downward facing dog.

Keep your head in a neutral position in line with your spine.

heels (see figure 4.21). Ensure that both your legs and arms are straight to lengthen your spine as far as possible.

CHEST STRETCH

Exercise Focus

Pectorals

Equipment

Swiss ball

How To

Kneel on the floor and place your forearm on a Swiss ball positioned to one side of your body. Keeping your shoulders parallel to the floor, drop your body downwards until you feel a stretch in your chest and

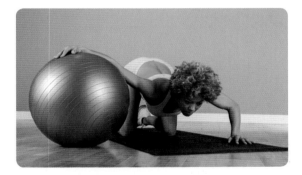

Figure 4.22   Chest stretch.

press your forearm into the Swiss ball (see figure 4.22). If you want to target your pectoralis minor (smaller muscle beneath the pectoralis major), place the front part of your shoulder, rather than your forearm, on the ball. Bend your elbow to 90 degrees and drop downwards into the stretch as before.

A small Swiss ball is preferable to allow you to square your shoulders to the ground most effectively.

NECK SIDE FLEXION

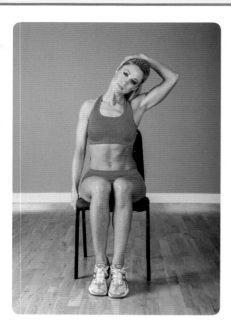

Exercise Focus

Neck

Equipment

Bench or chair

Keep your chin up and look straight ahead.

How To

Sit on a bench or chair with good upright posture. Grip onto the underneath of the bench or chair with one hand and lean away until you feel a stretch in your neck. Use your opposite hand to gently move your head away from your anchored shoulder (see figure 4.23).

Figure 4.23   Neck side flexion.

RHOMBOIDS STRETCH

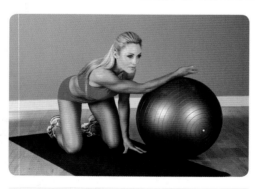

Figure 4.24   Rhomboids stretch.

Exercise Focus

Upper back

Equipment

Swiss ball

How To

Kneel next to a Swiss ball and place your farthest elbow on the ball and the hand of the other arm on the floor or the side of the ball for support. Move the arm on the ball across your body, keeping your elbow rested on the ball and your chest facing forwards. Press your elbow into the ball and allow your shoulder blade to move away from your spine (see figure 4.24).

Experiment with a different angle at your elbow to find the perfect stretch position for you.

FOUR-POINT GROIN STRETCH

Exercise Focus

Adductors

How To

Assume a kneeling position and spread your knees apart as far as you comfortably can. Reach forwards and place your hands on the floor in front of you. Push your hips towards the floor, keeping your back flat and chest up (see figure 4.25).

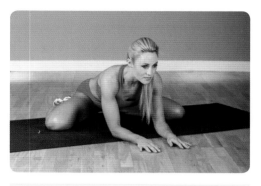

Figure 4.25   Four-point groin stretch.

This stretch is best performed with a contract–relax procedure, whereby you alternate pushing your body into the stretch and then relaxing out of it.

ILIOTIBIAL BAND WALL STRETCH

Exercise Focus

Iliotibial band

Equipment

Wall

How To

Stand sideways on and holding onto a wall or chair for support. Cross your inside leg over your outside leg and press your hip away from the wall or chair keeping your outside leg straight and your inside leg bent (see figure 4.26). To increase the stretch, bring your hips forwards slightly and rotate your pelvis toward the front.

Keep both feet flat on the floor throughout the stretch.

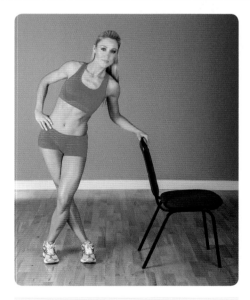

Figure 4.26   Iliotibial band wall stretch.

Stage 3: Recovery Methods

Specific recovery methods are useful following enduring and high-intensity sessions to speed up your recovery time (especially when training frequency is high) and for times when you are suffering with a particular tightness or injury.

Foam Rolling

Your muscles are surrounded by superficial fascia, a soft layer of connective tissue around the muscle. This layer is susceptible to damage and tightness during exercise, as well as injury through lack of stretching and in times of disuse, as the fascia and underlying muscle tissue become stuck together and form an adhesion. This adhesion will feel as though you have a knot in your muscles. It can reduce your muscle movement and flexibility, and can sometimes cause soreness.

Foam rolling is commonly used to release the tension in the fascia. The process of doing so is called myofascial release. This body-work technique uses gentle sustained pressure on the soft tissues whilst applying traction to the fascia. This softens and lengthens the fascia, and also breaks down any scar tissue or adhesions that may have built up. Through the technique of myofascial release, foam rolling can have the same beneficial effects as a sports massage, but it is available to you instantly and with much less cost. As they are usually made of simple polystyrene material, foam rollers are inexpensive and portable.

For effective foam rolling, simply follow these steps:

1. Place the foam roller on the floor and position the body part you wish to target on top of it.
2. Use the rest of your body to move the roller along the length of the muscle.
3. When you find a spot that is particularly tight, hold the position and apply greater pressure in that area until the tightness begins to ease.
4. Continue to move over the roller until the length of the muscle feels free of tension.

With some experimentation, you can target most muscle groups. To help get you started, figure 4.27 shows various main body parts to target with a foam roller.

Start with no more than 1 minute of rolling per body part, even if the tension does not completely ease during this time, to avoid inflammation or aggravation. With regular practice, your muscles will respond faster to this technique and you will be able to tolerate more pressure.

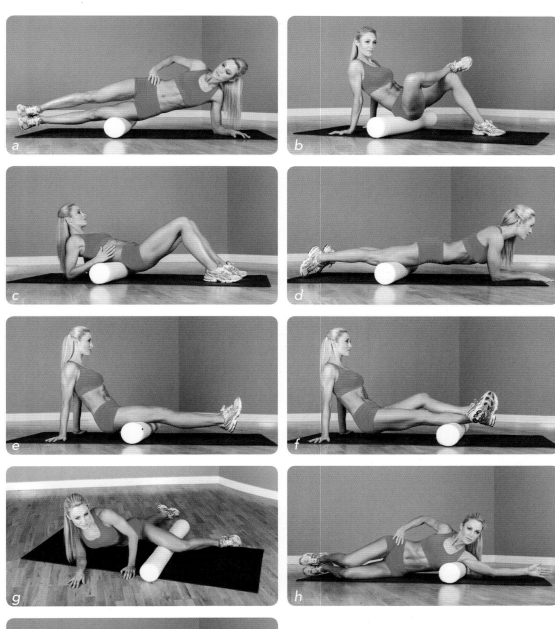

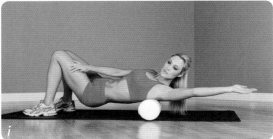

Figure 4.27 Foam Rolling Target Areas: *(a)* Iliotibial band, *(b)* glutes, *(c)* erector spinae, *(d)* quadriceps, *(e)* hamstrings, *(f)* calves, *(g)* adductors, *(h)* latissimus dorsi, and *(i)* shoulder girdle.

Sports Massage

A sports massage is a more mechanical and intricate way to achieve myofascial release, as the masseur will be able to use a smaller surface area (fingers and hands) to apply the pressure. Sports massage also serves a number of additional functions. The ongoing and extended pressure of massage increases blood flow and therefore muscle temperature, helping to increase flexibility and range of motion. Many psychological benefits to regular sports massage have been reported. Athletes claim it helps to relax them after a hard session and enhances their mind–body connection. Find a well-qualified masseur whose technique and approach works for you.

Ice Bath and Contrast Water Bath

Stepping into an ice bath is common practice amongst athletes to recover faster and reduce muscle soreness following intense training or competition. It works by constricting blood vessels and flushing out toxins, such as lactic acid, from the affected tissues. An ice bath may also reduce swelling and tissue breakdown. When you step out of the ice bath, your body begins to warm again and blood flow and circulation increase, aiding the healing process. More research needs to be done on the perfect protocol for maximising the benefits of an ice bath for recovery, but general guidelines are as follows:

- *Water temperature*: 12 to 15 degrees Celsius
- *Submersion time*: 5 to 10 minutes
- *Frequency*: Following intense training sessions

If you don't have an ice bath facility at your training centre, you can easily create your own. Simply fill your bath to hip level with cold water and add lots of ice. Submerge yourself immediately. You may not be able to achieve a water temperature as low as 12 degrees, but there is evidence that even cold-water immersion (around 24 degrees Celsius) can be just as effective (and far less daunting!).

VIBRATION TRAINING FOR WARMING UP AND COOLING DOWN

Vibration training with a machine such as a Power Plate uses acceleration and destabilisation to improve the strength and flexibility of your muscles. As you perform your exercises on the vibrating platform, which moves primarily up and down and commonly at a frequency of between 30 and 50 Hertz, your muscles detect the vibration and respond automatically to either contract or relax as a reflex action. This process occurs very quickly, acting to accelerate several responses in the body, making it a highly effective way to exercise, warm up and cool down. Performing your stretching exercises on a vibration platform can enhance the effects of your stretch as follows:

- Increases blood flow so the muscles become warmer more quickly, therefore reducing time required for stretching.
- Stimulates the Golgi tendon organs (GTOs) to switch on more quickly to induce muscle relaxation through a process known as autogenic inhibition.
- Increases the production of hormones, and speed of their delivery around the body, namely endorphins, testosterone and human growth hormone, to enhance exercise performance and strength development.
- Speeds up the delivery of oxygen and nutrients to the muscles for energy, recovery and repair.
- Reduces the amount of time required to perform the exercises as muscles respond to vibrations at an accelerated rate.

Simply hold (static) or move through (dynamic) your stretch position on the vibrating platform for up to 30 seconds per stretch, with your machine set at a frequency of 30 Hertz and low amplitude on a Power Plate machine.

To enhance and speed up your postexercise recovery, you can also perform massage exercises on the vibration platform. Simply lay your chosen body part on the platform and manoeuvre until the vibration targets any tight adhesive areas. You can achieve myofascial release in this way at speeds much faster than a masseur's hands can work. Perform each massage exercise for up to 60 seconds with your machine set at 40 to 50 Hertz and at a high amplitude on a Power Plate machine.

Alternatively you may like to try a contrast water bath, whereby you alternate between hot and cold baths. Common practice here involves 1 minute in a cold bath (12 to 15 degrees Celsius) and 2 minutes in a hot tub (37 to 40 degrees Celsius), repeated about 3 times. The principle here is that your blood vessels constrict and dilate rapidly as you move from cold to hot, further speeding up circulation and healing. A similar effect can be achieved in a shower alternating cold and hot temperatures.

AT A GLANCE

- The main purpose of a warm-up is to prepare your body for action. It can be broken down into 4 distinct stages: (1) cardiorespiratory exercise to increase your heart rate and temperature of your body, blood and muscles, (2) dynamic stretching to increase ROM around your joints, as well as flexibility and blood flow, (3) exercise drills that transition your now warmed muscles into the workout or sport you are about to perform, and (4) mental preparation to create the perfect state for you and your activity.

- The cool-down returns your body to its resting state and reduces the chances of muscle soreness. It has 3 main stages: (1) cardiorespiratory exercise that prevents blood pooling immediately after exercise by keeping a light blood flow to remove toxins, (2) static stretching while your muscles are warm and pliable, allowing you to achieve a deeper stretch, realign muscle fibres and establish your normal ROM, and (3) recovery methods such as ice baths and massage to speed up your recovery.

- Performing your stretching and massage exercises on a vibration platform has been found to increase blood flow and reduce the time required to both stretch and relax the muscles.

5

All In Aerobics

Aerobic training, whether you are familiar with the term or not, is what the majority of women do when they hit the gym for their cardio workouts, typically including running or cycling at a steady-state fixed pace. By providing the essential fitness base for participation in sport and burning significant amounts of calories that assist in weight-management efforts, aerobic workouts are invaluable in helping to maintain and improve our health and physiological functions. Health-related benefits of aerobic training include the following:

- Strengthens the heart muscle, improving its efficiency
- Improves circulation, so reducing blood pressure
- Enhances capability of the respiratory muscles
- Burns stores of fat, improving body composition
- Reduces the risk of diabetes
- Positively affects mental health, reducing the risk of depression

In addition, aerobic training has several performance-related benefits:

- Improves the ability to utilize fats, which are a rich energy source
- Increases the speed at which muscles recover from high-intensity exercise
- Enhances the blood flow through the muscles
- Increases the speed at which the aerobic system kicks in

But do you understand the principles behind this type of training and the different aerobic training methods available to you? Let's first understand exactly what aerobic training is and how it works, and then provide some fresh examples for you to try.

PHYSIOLOGY OF AEROBIC TRAINING

Aerobic capacity is the measure of how efficiently your lungs take in oxygen, your heart pumps it around your body in the bloodstream and your muscles then absorb and use it to generate movement. You will not be surprised to learn, therefore, the word *aerobic* translates literally to mean 'with oxygen'. Also known as stamina, cardiorespiratory fitness, endurance and staying power, the number of labels reflects its importance as both a key indicator of health status and a predictor of sporting performance. To help you understand the role of this biological process so you can tailor your training to improve aerobic capacity, let's investigate the physiology, beginning with respiration.

Mechanics of Breathing

When you inhale, your diaphragm contracts to move downwards; at the same time, the intercostal and pectoralis minor muscles pull the ribs up and out. This results in an increase in the volume in the thoracic cavity, decreasing the pressure within the chest. Due to the pressure gradient, air naturally flows from the area of higher pressure (the atmosphere) to the area of low pressure in the chest through the nostrils and mouth. It travels down the voice box and then the windpipe, which divides into two bronchial tubes that in turn subdivide to feed the lobes of the lungs. Obviously this is where the air eventually ends up. As we exhale, the whole pattern is reversed.

You may be surprised to learn the lungs are lopsided, with the right one comprised of three balloonlike lobes and the left made up of only two. The bronchial tubes split further into bronchioles and then further still into tiny air sacs, known as the alveoli. Blood enters the lungs via the pulmonary arteries, which split into smaller arterioles and then into the capillaries that form a network around the alveoli. This is where oxygen is taken up by the red blood cells and carbon dioxide is offloaded into the air to be expelled. Water is also removed from the body at this stage, since it is another waste product that results from the breakdown of glucose to fuel exercise. The oxygen-rich blood then flows out of the alveolar capillaries, through the venules and back to the heart via the pulmonary veins.

Blood Flow

The heart pumps oxygenated blood through the arteries to deliver this vital fuel throughout the body, yet its design is very simple. Sitting beneath and just to the left of the breastbone, it is a little larger than a tennis ball. The heart muscle itself, the myocardium, is divided into chambers that are separated by a smooth membrane. These chambers neatly sit on top of each other, with two on each side. The upper ones, known as atria, receive blood and then pass it on to the lower ones, called ventricles. Blood first enters the right atrium. Since it's returning from the body, it has given up its oxygen for the muscles to use, so it's low in oxygen concentration but high in carbon dioxide, the waste product it has removed from the tissues. Blood drains to the right ventricle, and is then pumped to the lungs via the pulmonary artery, which branches into two legs to serve each lung. The oxygenated blood returns to the heart by entering the left atrium. From there, it's shifted to the left ventricle, ready to be pumped through the aorta to the rest of the body. A break in continuous blood flow could be fatal, so the heart valves ensure blood is always moving in the right direction. The opening and closing of the valves generates the lub-dub noise that gets picked up by a stethoscope.

The whole cardiac cycle takes around only 0.8 seconds. Heart problems can be identified via a disruption in this cycle, as the pattern will change if the heart does not receive adequate supply of oxygen. When you take your pulse, you're actually measuring the number of cycles in a set period. Although 75 beats per minute is accepted as the average, fitter individuals tend to have a pulse of around 55. This variation is a result of the heart becoming stronger with regular exercise, and thus more able to pump out more blood with each beat. More blood with each beat means that the heart doesn't need to work as hard or pump as frequently, so is likely to last a lot longer than an organ under constant stress.

Now let's consider the essential transport system, the blood vessels that take oxygen to your exercising muscles. We have already seen that blood is ejected from the heart with some force into the arteries, so they have to have elastic walls that can stretch. This is important, as the recoil after they have expanded causes a squeezing effect that moves the blood through the network. When the arteries reach your muscles, they split into smaller vessels with thinner walls, called arterioles, and then again into even smaller capillaries. Their small size allows the vessels to get as close as possible to the tissues they serve, allowing them to deliver oxygen and remove carbon dioxide. This happens through a simple process of diffusion through the capillary walls, which is why they must be so thin. From here, the vessels begin their return journey, enlarging to form venules and then again to become veins, carrying carbon dioxide back to the heart. From there, it can be shifted to the lungs to be exhaled. Haemoglobin changes colour to red when carrying oxygen to the tissues and then to blue when transporting carbon dioxide away. This is seen most notably in the blue veins in the wrists. The arteries are not visible, as they are located deeper down.

Let's now apply the science of energy systems to establish the best way to achieve weight loss or, more specifically, fat loss. Now, a big word of warning here—weight-management programmes that set out to prioritise fat burning often advise doing continuous training below your anaerobic threshold threshold (anaerobic threshold being the point at which lactic acid builds up and leads to fatigue; more about this in chapter 6). Cardio equipment in gyms usually has a fat-burning-zone programme that alters effort level automatically if you exceed a working heart rate of around 55 to 65 percent of maximum. This is justified by the equipment manufacturers on the basis that maximal ratios of fat burning to glucose burning will be in place. This is true in terms of pure percentages, but at higher intensities, a greater number of total calories (and therefore more fat) will be burned for the same workout duration, even though it will be a smaller percentage of that total.

The argument against working at higher intensities is that there is a danger of exceeding the anaerobic threshold and therefore decreasing the percentage of fat burned in relation to carbohydrate. In addition, these intensities cannot be sustained for a long duration. These considerations are valid, but in order to maximise fat burning, you need to burn as many total calories as you can during the workout and to enhance your postexercise calorie burn. The bottom line is that working at higher intensities maximises calorie burning and results in your body continuing to burn more calories in recovery; therefore, you should tackle higher workloads during your workouts. Even if these higher workloads can only be sustained for 30 to 60 seconds before returning to lower work rates, it will still increase the total number of calories expended. Exceeding the anaerobic threshold will not stop fat burning; it will simply make a lower contribution to energy generation at these higher levels. Chapter 6 covers anaerobic training for fat loss in greater detail.

If fat loss is your goal, then interval training is a very beneficial approach. To achieve optimum results, you should vary your training sessions. Pick and mix from the different formats mentioned later, avoiding the natural inclination to stick with your favourite.

Energy Provision

Adenosine triphosphate (ATP) is the chemical in your muscles that breaks down to produce energy and relies on the breakdown of carbohydrate, fat and protein (see chapter 3). Every biological process demands energy, and this can only be in the form of ATP, which is made up of adenosine and three phosphate groups. Since strong bonds exist between the phosphate groups, breaking one of them results in a release of energy. In a muscle cell, the breakdown of ATP results in mechanical work (i.e., a muscle contraction) and also heat. So now you know why you feel warmer when you exercise.

When you first begin to exercise, the demand for energy increases relatively quickly, using your body's store of ATP within a couple of seconds, so more fuel is needed to produce further ATP. ATP can be resynthesised in three different ways, which are referred to as your body's energy systems. The first two energy systems are referred to as anaerobic and the third is known as aerobic. As we know from the beginning of this chapter, this implies that oxygen is present when ATP is being regenerated to keep you on the move.

In the presence of oxygen, fat can be used as a fuel to make ATP. Fat can't be used alone for ATP generation. Even when plenty of oxygen is present, there must always be a mixture of fat and glucose, hence the importance of carbohydrate in your diet. The aerobic phase of ATP generation takes place inside small cells called mitochondria that are particularly abundant within your slow-twitch muscle fibres (see chapter 7). These fibres have a considerable supply of capillaries bringing in oxygen that is then rapidly transferred to the mitochondria. Your fast-twitch muscle cells have a more limited capacity for aerobic work, although they can still do a little.

To help you to understand how the nature of your workout affects the results you will achieve, table 5.1 defines the differing intensities, with 1 being rest and 10 your maximum exertion.

Table 5.1   Effects of Different Effort Levels

Training zone	Intensity level 1–10	Results
General health	5–7	Increases utilisation of fat as a fuel, the number of mitochondria and the blood capillary density
Aerobic fitness	7–8	Improves recruitment of slow-twitch fibres, concentration of aerobic enzymes, oxygen transport and efficiency of glycogen (stored carbohydrate) utilisation
Anaerobic fitness	8–10	Improves recruitment of fast twitch fibres and muscle's ability to work without oxygen. This is covered in more detail in the next chapter.

UNDERSTANDING YOUR EFFORT LEVEL

Training intensity is often expressed as a percentage of $\dot{V}O_2$max. It is a measure of aerobic power, and specifically refers to the maximum amount of oxygen your body can process per kilogram of body weight per minute, as expressed in millilitres. Elite athletes tend to train at percentages of $\dot{V}O_2$max rather than at a percentage of maximum heart rate (HRmax) or effort level score because it has a greater relevance for controlled training adaptation. Some anaerobic training, such as circuit training, can improve your $\dot{V}O_2$max, but aerobic training has the biggest influence.

AEROBIC TRAINING METHODS AND EXERCISES

Now that you have a basic understanding of how we take in and transport oxygen, let's investigate the type of aerobic exercise you need to engage in to produce improvements in the cardiovascular and respiratory systems. Many formats exist, but here are a few that will improve fitness and sports performance.

Continuous Training

Continuous training is based on working out at a constant intensity for a specific duration of time. To do this, either in the gym or at home if you own cardio equipment, you can select the manual programme and maintain a set workload for however long you intend to exercise. This might be a certain speed or perhaps a resistance level. Clearly, a longer duration workout will require a lower intensity level to allow you to maintain the pace for the full duration. Similarly, do the opposite if you only have a short time period for your workout, as you'll be able to keep to the higher level if it's not for so long. Many advantages of this type of training exist, the most obvious being that it's simple and doesn't have sudden spikes in intensity that can cause discomfort. It has the great benefit of allowing you to monitor your progress, as you will soon notice that you are able to work at a higher speed or resistance and continue for longer. This might not be challenging enough for advanced exercisers, however; they could instead opt for light continuous training on their recovery days. Continuous training can also be performed outdoors with running or cycling for example, but note you will have less precise feedback about your pace and distance.

Continuous training is usually split into two types—less than 60 minutes and greater than 60 minutes. The shorter sessions are conducted at a moderate intensity, with the focus on burning calories. Endurance athletes will sometimes adopt this format, using a continuous pace but going at a much higher speed and referring to it as tempo training. The aim here is to exercise at an intensity close to their anaerobic threshold, the point at which the body begins to accumulate lactic acid in the muscles and fatigue sets in. The result of this training is an improvement in the body's ability to remove waste products, leading to better performance on race days.

Workouts longer than 60 minutes are known as long slow distance (LSD) or base sessions. They are ideal for endurance athletes seeking to improve their marathon or triathlon time. The benefits of this training include increases in the number of blood capillaries and the size of the mitochondria, which is where fat is mobilised as an energy source, so endurance improves and the body fuels from fat rather than carbohydrate. Care should be taken with this type of workout as it can lead to overuse injury, so the best way to follow this route is to mix different cardio modes to avoid too much of the same repetitive movement. In addition, dehydration is a genuine concern, so ingesting fluid at regular intervals is a must. Don't wait until you're thirsty to take a drink; take frequent sips of water or, ideally, an isotonic drink that can be quickly absorbed (see chapter 3).

Fartlek Training

Fartlek training is a phrase of Swedish origin that translates to mean speed play. It was developed by runners who changed their pace according to the surface they were running on, the gradient and just how they felt at a particular moment in time. Have fun with this format and introduce lots of variation. A bonus of this method is that it can easily be transferred to the pool and bike. Cardio machines usually incorporate a fartlek option, referred to as the random programme. If not, select the manual button and then change the speed, incline or resistance at irregular intervals.

Further advantages of this style of training include variety, to beat the boredom factor, and also development of different energy systems and muscle fibres due to the introduction of short, fast bursts. Being able to control the workout intensity, in that you can do more if you feel good and less if you're not having a great day, can lead to a more enjoyable exercise experience. However, one drawback is that you cannot compare workouts and measure your progress as easily. Since no two workouts are the same, you can't judge whether you're getting quicker or working harder.

Interval Training

Interval training consists of bouts of exercise interspersed with low-intensity periods to allow for recovery before the next effort increase. If the exercise is of very high intensity, the following period may even consist of complete rest, though we advise you always move around a little during this recovery to prevent potential blood pooling in the limbs, causing dizziness. True interval training differs from fartlek in that it features a set structure of work and rest periods. For example, performing a fast pace for 60 seconds followed by an easy pace for 30 seconds is labelled as a 2:1 work–rest ratio. Logically, when designing an interval workout, the higher the intensity is, the shorter the effort interval and the longer the rest period should be. A bout of 15 seconds of full-out sprinting might be followed by a slow pace of 45 seconds to give a 1:3 ratio. Cardio equipment always includes an interval, although sometimes it might be called the hill programme. If a built-in feature does not exist, select the manual setting and change the speed or resistance at the appropriate times.

Interval training allows you to do a considerable amount of high-intensity exercise, thus accelerating your results. It has the added flexibility of also being adaptable to anaerobic training (see chapter 6). You can push yourself in the work intervals, as your body will have time to rest immediately after, enabling lactic acid to be removed from the muscle cells and so reducing the discomfort that is associated with high-intensity exercise. Performing 10 sprints (either on foot or bike, or through the water) of 30 seconds with a 1-minute rest is quite manageable, and it accumulates to 5 minutes of maximal effort. However, if you simply set off on your sprint and try to maintain it for as long as possible, you will likely have to stop after around 2 minutes without achieving even half the volume of exercise in the first example. In addition, it's psychologically easier to work at higher intensities when you know there is a rest period coming. This is an ideal technique for guaranteeing that you continue to progress your fitness, as you can simply tweak the work-to-rest ratio.

Cross-Training

Cross-training refers to the practice of using different cardio modes on different days or even within the same workout. Options might include using the treadmill, rower and stationary cycle in the gym or, alternatively, jogging, cycling and swimming (think triathlon). The beauty of this approach is that it helps to relieve boredom by providing a changing stimulus and it also helps to reduce the risk of overuse injuries associated with repetitive movement patterns. In addition, since the different cardio exercises offer slightly different challenges, this method can lead to better balance in muscle development and better overall fitness gains.

If you're planning to complete a charity event involving one modality, it's better to prepare by training the actual discipline you will perform on the day, as cycling for a few weeks before taking the plunge to swim might leave you a few strokes short.

Negative Splits

Negative splits involve trying to complete the second section of an effort interval at a faster pace than the first portion. The interval might be split halfway, but the faster pace could also kick in three-quarters of the way through or even later. Negative splits will accustom you to changing pace. They are useful for preparing for races, as all distances over 400 metres will require you to speed up towards the finish.

Turnarounds

Turnarounds require you to complete repetitions of a set distance in a set time. The set time is usually quite generous, so you can decide either to take it easy with a short recovery or to push your pace and then enjoy a greater rest before your next repetition. For example, you could choose a distance of 400 metres and a time of 3 minutes. Select your own pace to run the distance. The faster you run to complete the 400 metres, the more time you will have to rest before beginning the next bout of effort. The slower you run, the less rest time you will have before the next interval begins. Turnarounds can be tailored to suit any level of fitness by manipulating the distance and time variables, but they particularly suit fitter women who have a competitive attitude. Manipulating the time and distance parameters enables you to increase the intensity, so this technique can also be used for anaerobic training (see chapter 6).

TIPS FOR BETTER TECHNIQUE

Since the primary training modes to improve your aerobic fitness are gym cardio machines and outdoor modalities involving running, cycling and swimming, here are a few pointers to help you to get the most from your workouts. Remember, better technique will lead to better performance and that can only lead to one thing—better results.

Gym Cardio Stations

- On each interval at slow or moderate pace, the resistance or incline should be at a challenging level, requiring you to be at 75 percent effort. You can reduce this for the fast pace and sprint bouts to raise your strides, strokes, or revolutions per minute.

- Be aware of your posture. In particular, do not lean forward on the stair climber or elliptical trainer.

- Try to mix and match equipment stations, as this will lead to a greater calorie burn and more rounded fitness gains. Perhaps complete one full interval block on the cycle, then switch to treadmill for the next block and the elliptical trainer for the last repetition, for example.

Outdoor Modalities

- Select terrain suited to your workout needs, whether that be a smooth pathway for cycling, soft grass for minimising joint impact whilst running or water with minimal current if you are getting accustomed to outdoor swimming. Mix it up to challenge yourself further.

- Select appropriate gear (equipment, clothing and shoes) that will stand up to the outdoor elements.

Run

- Concentrate on each phase of the movement. Lift the toe, bring the heel to the backside, drive the knee through, extend the lower leg and then, finally, claw the foot back.

- Keep your head neutral, your shoulders back and down and your abdomen just slightly pulled in. Your neck should be reclined.

- Ensure that your arms drive through in the direction you are travelling and not side to side with the elbow, as if rocking a baby. Pumping the fists forward and the elbows backward is one of the keys to increasing speed, should you desire to do so, as arms drive the legs.

- It's wise to invest in cushioned shoes, as these will absorb shock that might otherwise wear down your ankle, hip and knee joints from repetitive impact. A comfortable fit should allow room for your toes to expand when jogging. Also opt for seamless socks to further reduce the risk of sore feet.

Cycle

- Set the saddle at hip height and the handlebars at a height to give you a hinged position at the hip, but not so much that you have to round your spine and bend forwards.
- A common mistake is to push hard on the pedals in a high gear when, ideally, you should try to spin your pedals, as this will prevent fatigue and strain on the knees. You should both push the pedals down with your quadriceps and then pull them up using your hamstring and calf muscles for most effective spinning. Also, try to release your feet and keep ankles in a neutral or comfortable position.
- When approaching a hill, anticipate the lowest gear you will need and then settle into a rhythm. Standing up on the pedals is a good way to relieve the boredom of tackling a big incline. Rocking side to side will also help.
- Hands do a lot of work in hanging on, so they could be prone to fatigue, even injury. To prevent this, change hand positions every 10 minutes or so.

Swim

- On the breaststroke, keep a streamlined position by lowering your head on each stroke, so that the water comes just above the eyebrows. Try to focus on three phases of leg movements: Curl up, kick and then snap the inner thighs together.
- Try not to windmill the arms when crawling. As you bring your arm forward, point your elbow to the ceiling, with your hand directly below the elbow as it enters the water. Aim to take a breath on every third stroke.
- To improve your backstroke, hold a floating device on your thighs with one hand and swap hands after each stroke. This will help you achieve a full movement. Also, try holding both hands on the float to develop your kick, which should come from the hip rather than the knee.

AT A GLANCE

- Aerobic capacity, stamina, cardiorespiratory fitness, endurance and staying power all refer to the same measurement of fitness—your ability to take in, transport and then use oxygen to generate continuous exercise.

- Aerobic exercise takes place at low to moderate intensities. It depends on the performance of the lungs, heart and circulatory system.

- To maximise fat loss, your training should focus on total calorie burn rather than on percentage from fat as a fuel source. As a rule of thumb, then, work as hard as you can for as long as you've got!

6

Go Anaerobic

Anaerobic quite simply means without oxygen, and anaerobic training consists of intermittent bouts of high-intensity exercise involving weight training, explosive plyometric exercises, speed, agility and interval training. Therefore, if you have ever performed a short sprint or an explosive exercise such as a squat thrust or a burpee, then you have experienced anaerobic exercise.

Anaerobic training is commonplace amongst sportswomen and athletes, as most competitive sports, with only a few exceptions, will require a fast burst of movement at some point. For example, gymnasts, track sprinters, jumpers and throwers perform single maximal sprints or exertions, whilst team players in sports such as lacrosse, hockey and netball perform repeated bouts of high-intensity efforts. Even a distance runner is required to make a sprint finish, therefore moving into anaerobic mode. As such, all athletes train their anaerobic system to a greater or lesser degree depending on their sport's requirements. But anaerobic training is not just confined to athletes. Every female exerciser can reap the many rewards that anaerobic training can bring, from performance benefits to weight loss and exercise variety. First we want to explain a little more about the physiology of anaerobic training, and then we will move onto the benefits it can bring and the different methods used to achieve it.

PHYSIOLOGY OF ANAEROBIC TRAINING

The physiology of anaerobic training refers to the energy systems at work during this type of exercise and the different levels of adaptation that occur as a result. We will explore both here.

Anaerobic Energy System

The anaerobic energy system can be divided into two stages of energy contribution. The first stage is the use of the phosphagen system, known as the alactic stage, which lasts up to 10 seconds. The second is the glycolytic system, or the lactic stage, which can last up to 2 minutes.

Phosphagen System

The phosphagen system has no reliance on oxygen. Instead, it relies on stored energy sources (creatine phosphate) in your muscles and a chemical reaction that fires it up to produce energy in the form of adenosine triphosphate (ATP). An example of exercising using this system would be a 40-metre maximal sprint or lifting a set of heavy weights, and the first 10 seconds of any activity relies on the phosphagen system. Training this system allows you to generate maximal power for a short period of time, but it does require full recovery (e.g., 5 to 7 minutes of rest between sets or efforts) to fully regenerate the phosphagen and allow a subsequent maximal intensity effort to be performed effectively.

Glycolytic System

The glycolytic system also supplies your body with high powered energy and it can do so for up to 2 minutes, but it increasingly relies on oxygen contribution. Stored glucose is broken down by enzymes into pyruvic and lactic acids with the release of energy (ATP). To train this system, you need to exercise at a fast but not flat-out pace. It is commonly trained through intervals that range from 80 to 600 metres (when running is the modality of choice) with short recoveries. Fatigue is ultimately brought about by the production of the lactate and hydrogen ions, the body's protection mechanism at these intensities.

WEIGHT-LOSS TIP If your goal is to lose body fat and become leaner, anaerobic training can be a more effective way to do so than aerobic training due to the increase in highly metabolic muscle that develops and the "afterburn effect" that follows the workout

Physiological Adaptations to Anaerobic Training

Anaerobic training brings about physiological adaptations to the nervous, muscular, endocrine and cardiovascular systems that enable you to improve your athletic performance. Encouragingly, a number of these adaptations take place after just 4 weeks of including anaerobic training in your programme. Here are some performance improvements you can expect from regular anaerobic training.

Muscular Strength

Improvements are evident after just 4 weeks of heavy resistance training. Effects depend on the type of exercise and its intensity and volume. The more highly trained you are, the greater intensity and volume you will require for adaptations to continue. Improvements in muscular strength will set a great foundation for your body to improve at all sports and activities.

ENERGY PATHWAYS

Energy pathways all contribute towards the provision of a useable form of chemical energy called ATP, which is used to fuel the muscles for exercise. All energy pathways are active at the beginning of exercise. However, the contribution from each pathway will depend on the individual athlete, the effort applied and the rate at which energy is used. Here are some of the products essential in the production of energy from different systems:

- *Adenosine triphosphate (ATP)*—This complex chemical compound is formed with the energy released from food and stored in all cells, particularly muscles. Only from the energy released by the breakdown of this compound can the cells perform work. The breakdown of ATP produces energy and ADP.

- *Creatine phosphate (CP)*—This chemical compound stored in muscle aids in the manufacture of ATP when broken down. The combination of ADP and CP produces ATP.

- *Lactic acid (LA)*—This fatiguing metabolite of the glycolytic system results from the incomplete breakdown of glucose. Protons (the hydrogen ions) produced at the same time are thought to be responsible for restricting further performance. As the lactic acid and protons build up through greater exercise intensity, the accumulation makes further exercise harder and eventually impossible. This is essentially when your lactate threshold is reached. The more intense your exercise intervals or efforts, the greater the concentration of lactate build-up.

- *Oxygen (O_2)*—In aerobic running, ATP is copiously manufactured from food, mainly carbohydrates and fat. This is the prime energy source during endurance activities (see chapter 5 for more information).

Power

Increased force output at higher velocities and increased rate of force development is improved following power training (a form of anaerobic training that utilises the phosphate energy system). This is great if you partake in a sport or activity involving jumping, throwing or any other explosive action.

Local Muscular Endurance

This is enhanced by training your body in the lactic stage of energy contribution with short sprint repetitions and short recoveries or with longer efforts up to 600 metres and longer recoveries. This type of training improves your oxidative capacity through increased metabolic enzyme activity and mitochondrial and capillary numbers, as well as improved buffering capacity and muscle fibre-type transitions. In short, these improvements mean delaying the pain and discomfort caused by the accumulation of lactic acid, thus enabling you to maintain your effort for longer, a great benefit for those speed endurance gym sessions and track, rowing, cycling and swimming performances.

Aerobic Capacity

Circuit training and other sessions involving high volume workloads and short recoveries have been shown to increase $\dot{V}O_2$max. Additionally, heavy resistance training using an anaerobic protocol can also improve aerobic capacity in deconditioned individuals.

Motor Performance

These are improvements to the movement pattern involved in the exercise and are based on the specificity of the exercises or modalities performed. Resistance training has been shown to increase running economy, vertical jump, sprint speed, swinging and throwing velocity and kicking performance, all of which are beneficial to both the professional athlete and regular exerciser.

ANAEROBIC TRAINING AND WEIGHT LOSS

Although it is commonly assumed that exercising below your anaerobic threshold is optimal for weight loss or, more specifically, fat loss (see previous chapter), this conclusion does not take into account the physiological adaptations from anaerobic training that enhance calorie burn and fat loss or the excess energy requirements that follow anaerobic training.

Resistance training, one form of anaerobic training, increases lean tissue mass, daily RMR and energy expenditure during exercise, helping you to become leaner and more efficient at fat burning. What's more, the energy requirement following anaerobic training to repair muscle tissue and replace energy stores is greater than that required after aerobic training. Consequently, your body continues to burn more calories during your recovery. This is known as the "afterburn effect."

Hormonal Response

Anaerobic exercise, especially resistance exercise, has been found to elevate testosterone, growth hormone and cortisol for up to 30 minutes post exercise. This effect is more pronounced in men, but it can also be found in women. These testosterone increases can produce greater strength development and consistent resistance training leads to chronic changes and the ability to exert more effort in successive training sessions.

ANAEROBIC TRAINING METHODS AND EXERCISES

Anaerobic training methods include resistance exercises for strength development, plyometric and sprint exercises for power training, agility exercises and intervals. We will focus here on interval training, as exercises for the other methods are covered extensively in the other chapters of this book. Check out chapter 7 for strength exercises, chapter 8 for power training examples and chapter 9 for agility movements.

Interval training is a great method of cardiorespiratory training that particularly develops anaerobic fitness, whether you are a sportswoman or recreational exerciser. It can be carried out on any piece of cardio equipment—treadmill, bike or elliptical machine—as well as on the track, road, field and in the swimming pool, and can be tailored to different levels of fitness and to different training goals. Interval training includes performing your chosen activity for a specific distance or time and exercising to a designated heart rate, rating of perceived exertion (RPE), HRmax or $\dot{V}O_2$max percentage. The interval can be as short as 6 seconds or as long as 20 minutes and can have a primarily aerobic or anaerobic affect. Examples of aerobic interval training can be found in chapter 5: All In Aerobics.

For anaerobic development, the maximum interval time is likely to last around 60 seconds. The recovery for interval training can be passive or active, and it takes place at the end of each completed interval. A passive rest involves walking or standing around for a set time after the completion of each interval. Despite its name, we do not advise you simply flop down on the floor during this time! Simple walking and passive stretching will maintain your physiological readiness for the next interval and help keep blood flowing to remove the toxins that have accumulated. Active recovery involves a set period of gentle cardiorespiratory work between your more intense intervals, such as a light jog or continued pedal turnover at a lighter resistance if cycling. Interval training sessions can be of a low, medium or high intensity. We will focus here on the medium- to high-intensity sessions to elicit the anaerobic training adaptations described.

The benefits of interval training, in addition to improving aerobic and anaerobic fitness, include the following:

- You can reduce your exercise time as the overall intensity is higher, meaning you get fit and burn calories faster in this more condensed time.
- It removes boredom associated with steady-state exercise, as you focus on one interval, or effort, at a time. This has an additional motivational factor in making the session seem more manageable and the achievements more noticeable.
- The recovery periods require your cardiovascular system to continue to work to return your body to a more rested physiological state, once again increasing the total workload and calorie burn, as well as improving fitness further.
- It increases lactic acid tolerance.
- It helps avoid injuries associated with repetitive overuse, common in endurance athletes, and increases training intensity without overtraining or burnout.
- Variety in the different interval sessions you can incorporate into your programme ensures that exercise stays fun and challenging and that your body continuously adapts. Your body responds best to change and variety.

You can choose from numerous interval training sessions. It is fun and easy to make up your own. Here are the interval training variables you can adapt to suit your training level and exercise goals:

- Duration (time/distance) of intervals
- Duration of rest/recovery phase
- Number of repetitions of intervals
- Intensity (speed) of intervals
- Frequency of interval workout sessions
- Modality of interval
- Progression (Don't try to progress all variables at the same time!)

Now, we will outline a selection of sample interval training workouts for developing your anaerobic fitness. The full workout details can be found in chapter 11.

INTERVAL TRAINING SAFETY AND CONSIDERATIONS

Anaerobic style interval training requires you to work at a moderate to high intensity of exercise, so it is important to be fully prepared and conditioned as follows to maximise your enjoyment and results:

- Always warm up before beginning your interval training session (see chapter 4 for ideas) as high-intensity training (HIT) characteristics of interval training will require maximal muscle recruitment.

- Only perform HIT intervals once a suitable base of cardio-respiratory fitness has been established.

- Stop the interval session when you can no longer maintain form and when your interval times show a noticeable decline.

- Aim to bring your heart rate down to 100 to 110 bpm during the recovery phase.

- Perform HIT intervals an average of two times per week to see adaptations after 4 weeks of training. Combine with other forms of anaerobic training (resistance, power and agility) as well as aerobic training to develop all-round fitness and to improve performance.

- Consider specificity of the interval training you practice—do the modality and intervals mimic your own sport and recreational requirements? This is essential for transfer of training to performance.

- If injured, consider performing low- to medium-intensity intervals, changing modality (from running to bike or pool if impact is a problem) and doing more aerobic exercise, as well as specific rehab. Always consult your physician or physiotherapist if you are unsure if you should perform HIT intervals.

- Remember to breathe! It is not uncommon for those new to anaerobic training to hold their breath during a sprint effort. This will only act to enhance lactic generation and fatigue. Breathe naturally, not forcefully, during intervals.

- Record your training sessions in your diary so that you can apply progressive overload to make gains at the right rate. See chapter 10 for more details on programme design and chapter 12 for information on creating a training diary.

BACK-TO-BACK 60-METRE RUNNING SPRINTS

Mark out 60 metres and sprint back and forth between the markers, resting for 10 to 20 seconds between each effort. Perform multiple reps and sets. This type of session relies on fast regeneration of ATP and therefore trains your phosphagen system. The rest between sets is considered long enough to recover 90 percent peak power output, enabling you to perform subsequent sets at close to the same speed as the previous one.

INCLINE TREADMILL SPRINTS

Stand on the edge of the treadmill (i.e., off the moving belt) and bring the treadmill up to your starting speed and gradient. Step onto the moving belt and sprint. After 30 seconds, step off the belt onto the edges of treadmill for 30 seconds of recovery, and then repeat subsequent sprints. This session relies on fast regeneration of ATP and therefore trains your phosphagen system. The incline will also encourage greater glute activation and require more work from your calf and quadricep muscles.

WEIGHT-LOSS TIP Sprinting with an incline or up a hill will increase your calorie burn, as it increases the intensity of each sprint effort and recruits a greater number of muscle fibres. A direct correlation exists between intensity and calories burned.

BIKE SPRINT EFFORT SESSION

Perform a series of sprint efforts—60 seconds, 45 seconds, 30 seconds and 15 seconds—with a recovery equal in time to the next effort to be performed. Once you have completed one set, continue straight into the next one, building up the number of sets you can complete from week to week. This session will tax your glycolytic system. The active recovery advised will encourage faster removal of this lactic acid produced and will pay back the oxygen debt that has accrued during the interval. Cycling is often a quadriceps-dominant exercise modality for many, but a more efficient technique whereby you actively claw your heel to your bottom during the recovery phase of the cycle will encourage greater activation of your calves and hamstrings.

TRACK SPRINT PYRAMID SESSION

Sprint distances of 200 metres, 250 metres, 300 metres and repeat in descending order back down to 200 metres, walking slowly for an active recovery of 3 to 5 minutes between sets. Ideally, you would sprint on a running track and at close to maximum speed for each distance. This session develops local muscular and speed endurance, helping your body to delay the onset of lactic acid and therefore achieve faster times over these sprint distances. A grass surface can also be used if you mark out the distances to guide your session.

SPINNING SESSION

Cycle for 20 to 30 minutes, performing a sporadic number of efforts ranging from 10 to 60 seconds in duration, including hill climbs and hovers (where you slightly elevate your bottom above your seat). You determine the speed, time and type of effort as you see fit during the session. This session is based on early forms of interval training, known as fartlek, where the intervals are more casual and unstructured.

STAIR CLIMBS

Sprint up the stairs (30 to 50 steps), covering single, double or triple steps with each stride, and then jog slowly to the bottom. Repeat the process. Stair climbing is great for developing overall quickness and foot speed whilst getting a great workout.

SWIM SPRINTS

Swim predetermined distances between 25 and 50 metres, rest and repeat, increasing your number of repetitions from session to session. Train at close to your maximum swimming speed for your chosen stroke and distance.

AT A GLANCE

- Anaerobic training refers to training without oxygen and includes intermittent high-intensity bouts of exercise, such as weight training, explosive plyometric exercises, and speed, agility and interval training.

- Energy is provided for anaerobic training from the phosphagen system (in the first 10 seconds of exercise) and from the glycolytic system (for up to 2 minutes) of high-intensity exercise.

- Weight loss, particularly fat loss, can be accelerated by anaerobic training due to the resulting increase in lean muscle tissue, which increases metabolism and calorie burn during exercise, and the "afterburn effect," where the body works to recover and repair muscle tissue and repay the oxygen debt accrued after exercise, which requires additional calories.

- Interval training is the most common form of anaerobic training. It includes performing high-intensity exercise efforts interspersed with passive or active recovery periods. Interval training is suitable for professional sportswomen for improving performance and lactate tolerance and for recreational gym goers for improving fitness and performance and enabling controlled progression.

7

Going Strong

This chapter looks at muscular strength and local muscular endurance, investigating basic anatomy and how the muscles function in order to make sense of the different training modes proposed that will lead to gains in these areas. An obvious starting point is to define these two parameters, something that is easily explained using the strength–endurance continuum, an imaginary line with absolute strength at one end and pure endurance at the other. This illustrates that there exists no clear point at which strength training ends and endurance training begins; rather a gentle shift in emphasis occurs as we move along the line. So every workout format will improve both strength and endurance within the muscles; however, improvements could be quite minor for one of them, depending on the precise protocol adopted.

The important thing to know about strength training is it isn't just for performance sportswomen and gym bunnies. It's an incredibly useful weapon in your armoury in the pursuit of weight-loss goals. Here are a few reasons why:

- As with other modes of training, strength training burns calories, helping to achieve an end-of-day calorie deficit.
- Since women have lower testosterone levels than men, they do not grow big muscles a result of regular strength training. Rather, they will develop a lean, toned appearance.
- Studies show that after strength training, the metabolic rate remains elevated for a while, more so than after a cardio workout, again leading to a greater calorie burn.
- Strength training leads to increased lean tissue (i.e., muscle that has a higher resting metabolic rate than fat, for example). This brings the welcome bonus that you'll burn more calories, even when you're sleeping.

In order to fully appreciate the many performance and aesthetic benefits strength training can bring, it's really useful to first understand how the muscles are made up and how they respond to different workouts. Armed with this knowledge, you can better judge how to plan your workout schedule in order to achieve your specific goals.

STRENGTH AND MUSCLE STRUCTURE

Muscles are comprised of two distinct fibre types. This is a vital concept to grasp, as they respond differently to training stimulus and so determine our results. *Slow-twitch* muscle fibres are red in colour, as they hold myoglobin where oxygen is stored. They also contain a high concentration of mitochondria, an enzyme that is vital for the production of energy in the muscle cells. These muscle fibres are slow to contract, but also slow to fatigue. So, they are ideally suited to activities of a lower intensity and longer duration, in other words, endurance events. *Fast-twitch* muscle fibres are white in colour and contract quickly but also tire equally rapidly, so they are suited to high-intensity, short-duration exertions. Unlike the slow-twitch fibres, fast-twitch can be subdivided into two categories. Some fibres can contract quickly and have a little more staying power than typical fast-twitch fibres. These pink fibres, as they are known, are incredibly useful as they can assist the slow-twitch fibres if the intensity increases in an endurance event. They also support the fast-twitch fibres when they begin to fail, allowing for a few extra repetitions, yards or seconds. The percentage split of which fibre type you possess is genetically dependent, hence the suggestion that if you wish to win an Olympic gold medal, you should choose your parents and grandparents very carefully!

Following is a brief explanation of the different muscle fibres.

Type I

Type I (slow-twitch, slow-oxidative, aerobic, oxygen-burning) muscle fibres are fatigue resistant and have a high capacity for aerobic energy supply and a limited potential for explosive force production. Endurance athletes train their slow-twitch fibres, and they may naturally have more endurance fibres. Slow-twitch fibres have low force production, slow contraction speeds and high endurance. They are also aerobic. Therefore, they are not favoured during exercises requiring high power. Instead, they are used to keep our stability muscles active throughout to support the powerful movements.

Type IIa

Type IIa (fast-twitch, slow glycolytic, anaerobic, carbohydrate-burning) glycolytic muscle fibres can produce force rapidly. They have high anaerobic power, possess good aerobic and anaerobic potential, and have a greater resistance to fatigue than Type IIb fibres. They are therefore in demand when repeated powerful movements are performed.

Type IIb

Type IIb (fast-twitch, fast-glycolytic, anaerobic, carbohydrate-burning) glycolytic fibres have poor aerobic capacity and good anaerobic characteristics. They are therefore most suited for single powerful movements.

This understanding of muscle structure leads to the following training advice:

- Strength will be improved by stimulating the fast-twitch fibres, implying that you should lift heavy loads. By definition, then, this will allow for only a low number of repetitions. The body's adaptive response will be to enhance the neuromuscular processes that govern the number of muscle fibres recruited in the exercise together with how frequently they fire, so resulting in an increase in the force generated.

- Working with a moderate load allows a greater number of repetitions to be performed and results in both fast- and slow-twitch fibres being deployed. This taxes a greater number of muscle fibres, which develop by the thickening of the individual fibres, thus increasing their cross-sectional area. Therefore, this is the optimum route for improving muscle size.

- Endurance capacity will be heightened through adaptations in the slow-twitch fibres that respond to low resistance and high numbers of repetitions. Training for endurance gains carries an associated loss in strength and muscle mass. Although the slow-twitch fibres increase in size, they are much smaller than their fast-twitch counterparts.

This information enables us to set training guidelines to achieve specific goals, as shown in Table 7.1.

Table 7.1   Effects of Repetition and Load Variation

Number of repetitions	Resistance (as a % of 1-repetition maximum)	Primary result
1–5	85–100%	Increase in strength
6–8	75–85%	Increase in strength plus size
9–12	70–75%	Increase in size
13–20	60–70%	Increase in endurance

A key element here is to work with a resistance based on your one-repetition maximum (i.e., the amount of weight you can lift only once, with correct form, for each exercise in your routine). To discover your single repetition maximum, use our suggested 1 Rep Max test featured in chapter 2: Fitness Assessments. Alternatively, trial and error can help you identify appropriate weights to work with. The rule of thumb is that if the last couple of repetitions are difficult to complete, whether in the low-, mid- or high-repetition range, then the load is in the correct area.

KEYS TO MAKING PROGRESS

Resistance training actually breaks down the muscle at cellular level. In addition to this, the body undergoes adaptations by absorbing protein into the muscles to help them to repair. The genius here is a phenomenon at work known as supercompensation, whereby the muscles cleverly absorb protein more than is required to repair. So, the muscle fibres become thicker and therefore stronger. Since you will become stronger over time, if you're working out regularly, you will need to incrementally increase the loads you lift for each exercise. This is the principle of progressive overload. If you stick to the same weight you always use, the law of diminishing returns will apply and you will see very little improvement despite your continued endeavours. In addition, you can increase the intensity of your workout as you become stronger by performing extra sets of each exercise while slowing down the movement or reducing the amount of time you rest between each set. This results in the recruitment of more muscle fibres. A bonus side-effect of achieving muscular overload that is worthy of mention here is that it also helps to strengthen both the ligaments and tendons. It also stimulates an increase in bone mineral content through a phenomenon known as the piezoelectric affect (a significant factor in the prevention of osteoporosis). For more detail, see chapter 10.

RESISTANCE TRAINING METHODS AND EXERCISES

The beauty of resistance training is that, at the cellular level where the changes take place, your muscles have no way of identifying exactly which exercises you're doing or the tools being used. It actually doesn't matter as long as you hit fatigue on the last couple of repetitions. This is great news, as it allows you to choose from the wide spectrum of resistance modes on offer, ensuring your workouts are never boring.

Resistance Machine Exercises

Resistance machines are found in nearly every gym. They generally target a specific muscle or group of muscles with one exercise. They allow you to attempt heavy loads without the need for a spotter's assistance in assuming the start position, and also remove the likelihood that weights will drop on you (or worse, on others!). Range of movement is fixed, however, so the machine might not suit your body shape perfectly. The cost and size of these items pretty much rules them out of home use; thus, they are accessible to you only if you belong to a health club or leisure centre.

One simple routine is based on working the larger muscle groups first. The premise here is that you should tackle the most demanding exercises when you have lots of energy. Then, as you tire, the exercises for the smaller muscle groups are not so taxing. This is a sensible injury-prevention tactic. The following section outlines a sample programme that works the larger muscle groups first. Performing every exercise in the order listed will give you a great total-body workout in around 30 minutes if you aim for 1 set of each exercise. Clearly, if you're more advanced, you should aim for 2 or 3 sets of each exercise to ensure results by reaching momentary muscular fatigue.

LEG PRESS

Exercise Focus

Glutes, quadriceps and hamstrings

How To

Sit at the station in a comfortable position, with your upper body pressed against the back of the seat so that your back is fully supported by the backrest. Place both feet on the foot plate with your knees bent as far as is comfortable (see figure 7.1*a*). Push down on foot plate and fully extend your legs (see figure 7.1*b*). Slowly return to the original position, lowering the weight plates with control.

Be careful not to lock your knees at the end of the lift.

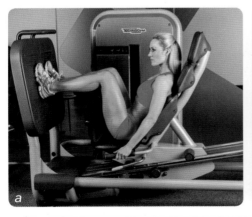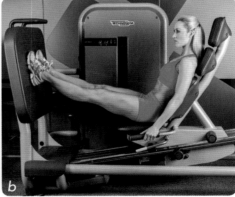

Figure 7.1   Leg press.

SQUAT

Exercise Focus

Glutes, quadriceps and hamstrings

How To

Stand inside the cage with the bar placed behind your neck, resting on your shoulders. Position your feet hip-width apart and the bar at a height that allows your legs to be straight but not locked out at the knees (see figure 7.2a). Firmly grip the bar at a position wider than shoulder width, and lift the bar from the cage and take the whole weight. Keeping your abdominal muscles pulled in tight, bend your knees and lower your backside (see figure 7.2b). Press through your heels to extend your legs and return to the standing position.

Your upper body will naturally hinge forward at the hip as you lower, but take care not to round your spine.

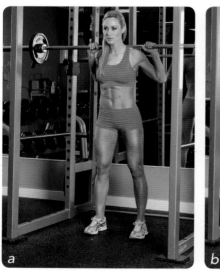 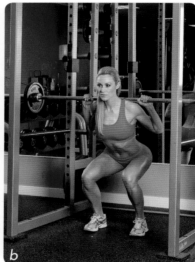

Figure 7.2   Squat.

CHEST PRESS

Exercise Focus

Pectorals, deltoids and triceps

How To

Sit on the seat with your feet flat on the floor, ideally at a height with the handles at chest level. Take hold of the handles and lift your elbows out to the side (see figure 7.3a). Keeping your shoulder blades drawn together, press the handles forward and fully extend the arms, but do not lock out your elbows (see figure 7.3b). Slowly return the weight to the start position.

Exhale on the exertion to add extra oomph to your effort.

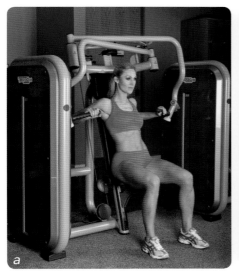 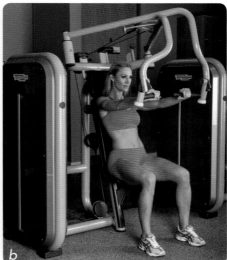

Figure 7.3   Chest press.

SEATED ROW

Exercise Focus

Upper back, latissimus dorsi, deltoids and biceps

How To

Sit with your chest placed against the rest at a height so you can comfortably reach the handles with your arms extended but not stretched (see figure 7.4a). Keeping your abdominals engaged and elbows high, draw your arms back (see figure 7.4b). Release slowly to lower the weight plates with control, and return to the start position.

Although the arms are moving, try to forget them. Focus instead on squeezing your shoulder blades together.

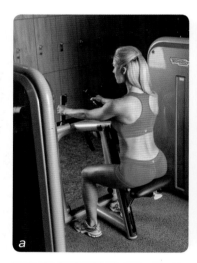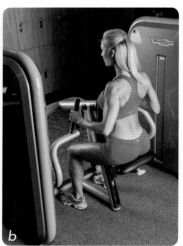

Figure 7.4   Seated row.

SHOULDER PRESS

Exercise Focus

Deltoids and triceps

How To

Sit with your back pressed firmly against the seat and your feet flat on the floor. Take the handles in line with your shoulders and move your elbows out to the side to open your chest (see figure 7.5*a*). Lift the handles up overhead in a smooth motion, taking care not to fully extend your arms (see figure 7.5*b*). Slowly lower to the start position.

As you lift, you may have an urge to arch your back. Concentrate on keeping your tummy pulled in.

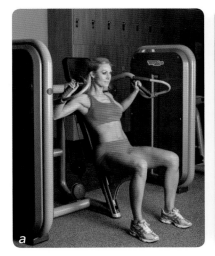 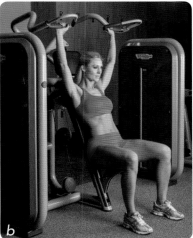

Figure 7.5   Shoulder press.

CABLE CURL

Exercise Focus

Biceps

How To

Stand facing the cable machine, holding the handle in front of the thighs with your arms extended and palms facing upwards (see figure 7.6a). In order to avoid your body swaying and potentially putting unwelcome strain on your lower back, place your feet slightly wider than hip width, keeping your knees soft and your abdominal muscles pulled in tight. Slowly bend the elbows to lift the bar up towards the chin but keep your elbows in contact with your ribs at all times and resist the temptation to swing your upper arm to assist the movement (see figure 7.6b). Lower the weight under control to the start position.

Concentrate on keeping your shoulders and upper arms fixed in position throughout the lift to ensure the whole effort (and therefore benefit) is associated with the biceps only.

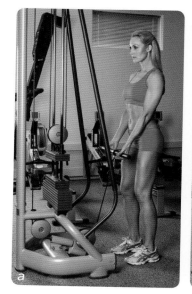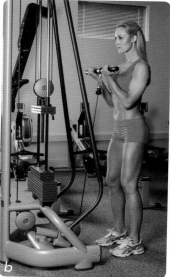

Figure 7.6   Cable curl.

TRICEPS PUSH-DOWN

Exercise Focus

Triceps

How To

Stand facing the cable machine, with knees slightly bent and abdominal muscles pulled in, and take the bar in an overhand grip at about shoulder width (see figure 7.7a). Keeping your elbows fixed by your side, press down on the bar to extend your arms (see figure 7.7b). Slowly bend the elbows to return to the start position.

Try to think about your triceps muscles contracting and shortening as you press down.

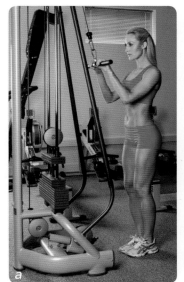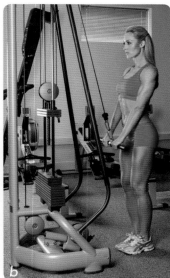

Figure 7.7   Triceps push-down.

ABDOMINAL CRUNCH

Exercise Focus

Abdominals and obliques

How To

Sit on the seat, take hold of the handles and place your feet behind the pads (see figure 7.8a). Focus on generating the movement by contracting your abdominal muscles rather than pulling with your arms. Squeeze down. Aim to squeeze your ribs to meet your hips (see figure 7.8b). Release gently to return to the start, but keep the tension on.

Visualise your abdominal muscles as a spring. Think of taking it in your hand and squeezing it so the ends come closer together.

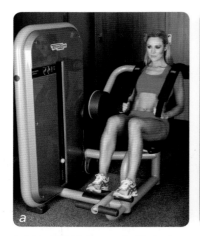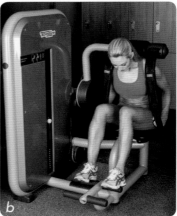

Figure 7.8   Abdominal crunch.

WHY WEIGHT?

Hydraulic resistance machines employ compressed air to remove the need for weights and plates and therefore remove the associated risk of injury. These machines have come a long way in terms of design. They now feature easy-to-adjust resistance levels and feedback regarding the resistance levels being used. Unlike weight and plate machines, however, you don't need one for each exercise, as most feature what is referred to as a dual positive motion (i.e., you have to push and pull in both directions, rather than lowering the weight against the force of gravity). So, although they are still relatively expensive, they will not take up as much space as fixed-weight machines. The dual positive movement removes the negative phase of the exercise, or the eccentric contraction whereby the muscle is under tension whilst lengthening, which has been shown to significantly reduce the effect of delayed-onset muscles soreness that follows an intense workout.

Free-Weight Exercises

Free weights might once have had the negative connotation of big beefy meatheads grunting loudly as they drop chunks of iron to the floor with a crash, but times have changed. Rusty bars and plates have now been replaced by soft-to-touch updates in vibrant colours, and weighted balls, kettlebells, ViPR and powerbags have been added to the mix. You can now lift, carry and throw a fabulous array of tools to improve your strength. Without doubt, you need a higher skill level than when working on fixed machines, and you might drop something on yourself, but these drawbacks are outweighed by the qualities of free weights: They are easily transportable, they occupy little storage space and they can be relatively inexpensive. Most importantly, they allow for a whole-body approach by demanding recruitment of fixator or stabilising muscles (e.g., the core muscles required to maintain good spinal alignment throughout specific exercises). In contrast to machines, free weights allow for more functional training (i.e., exercises that mirror movement patterns you use in particular sports or in everyday tasks).

A number of different workouts now follow, with each exercise illustrated and described in detail, to help you to master the technique. You can choose whether you wish to follow the whole routine or simply cherry-pick one or two exercises to add to your current workout.

Dumbbell Exercises

Following are several dumbbell exercises that you can choose to use in your workouts.

SQUAT LATERALS

Exercise Focus

Glutes and deltoids

How To

Stand tall with your feet hip-width apart and your shoulders drawn back. Hold the dumbbells by your side with your palms facing inward (see figure 7.10a). Keeping the weight in your heels and your chest lifted, bend your knees and push your backside behind you to descend into a squat. At the same time, lift your arms up to the side so the dumbbells end up just above shoulder level, remembering to keep your elbows slightly bent throughout (see figure 7.10b). As you contract your thighs to press up to a standing position again, slowly lower your arms.

Although you may be able to easily perform both the squat and the lateral raise, when combined, they exert a great demand on the core, so focus on keeping your centre tight.

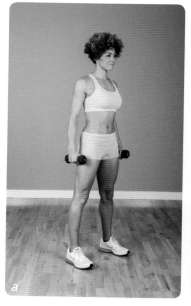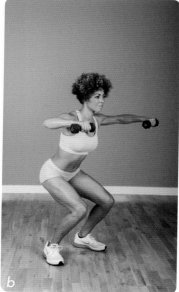

Figure 7.10   Squat laterals.

LUNGE SWING

Exercise Focus

Glutes, quadriceps, hamstrings, triceps and biceps

How To

Standing in a static lunge position, ensure your feet are not in line but are spread for balance. Bear your weight on the ball of your rear foot and keep it facing forward. To start, hold the dumbbell with one hand and place it behind your shoulder, keeping the elbow high (see figure 7.11a). Extend your arm to lift the dumbbell (see figure 7.11b) and then continue the motion by letting it swing forwards and down. Lower down into the lunge as far as is comfortable, but be wary not to bend the front knee beyond 90 degrees (see figure 7.11c). As you now swing the dumbbell forward and up to return to the start position, simultaneously contract your legs to lift out of the deep lunge. Repeat on the other arm with the opposite foot forward. Pull the abdominal muscles in tight to keep your back from arching and maintain a comfortable speed.

Do not let momentum take your arm into an extreme extended position. Concentrate on control through your shoulder girdle.

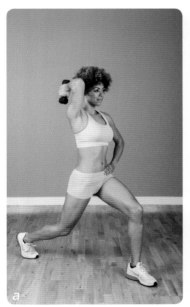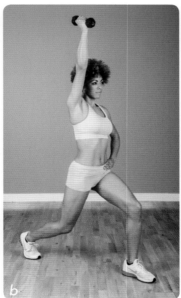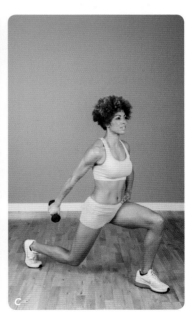

Figure 7.11   Lunge swing.

FLY

Exercise Focus

Pectorals and deltoids

How To

Lie on your back with your knees bent so you can place your feet flat on the floor. Hold the dumbbells directly above your chest, one in each hand, with your palms facing in and your elbows bent just a little (see figure 7.12a). Lower your arms to the side in an arc movement until the back of your upper arms touch the floor (see figure 7.12b) then raise them to the start position by squeezing your pectoral muscles.

Focus on pulling your tummy in throughout the movement to avoid being pulled into an exaggerated lumbar curve.

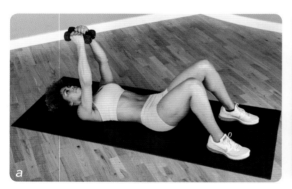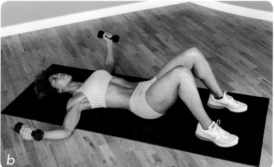

Figure 7.12   Fly.

BENT-OVER ROW

Exercise Focus

Upper back, deltoids and biceps

How To

Hold a dumbbell in each hand. With your feet slightly wider than hip-width apart and your knees soft, hinge forward at your hip, keeping a curve in your lower back and avoiding the temptation to round your spine. Extend your arms down towards the floor, but don't let the weight of the dumbbells pull your shoulders down (see figure 7.13*a*). You will really need to focus on your core muscles, pulling in your navel, from start to finish of this exercise. Bend your elbows to lift the weights and concentrate on squeezing your shoulder blades together to get the most benefit for the upper back muscles (see figure 7.13*b*).

Lift only as high as is comfortable. Do not alter your upper-body position.

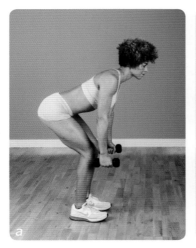 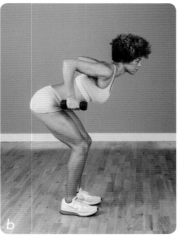

Figure 7.13   Bent-over row.

DUMBBELL WALKOUT

Exercise Focus

Abdominals and triceps

How To

Start on all fours, with the knees under the hips and the hands under the shoulders. Rest your hands on the dumbbells (see figure 7.14a). Keeping your spine in a comfortable position, with just a small curve in your lower back, walk your hands forwards one at a time (see figure 7.14b), then as far as you can until your hips begin to sag down (see figure 7.14c), then return by walking slowly back.

Engage the deep abdominal muscles and those around your shoulder blades to provide stability and prevent the dumbbells from rolling.

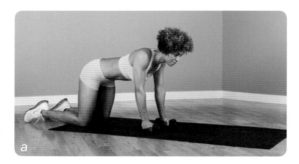

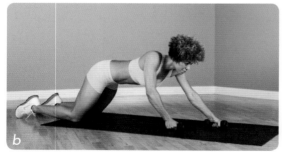 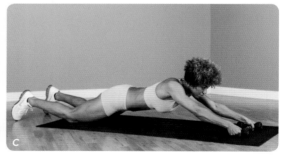

Figure 7.14   Dumbbell walkout.

RESISTED SIT-UP

Exercise Focus

Abdominals

How To

Start in your normal sit-up position, and then place either one or both dumbbells on your chest in a comfortable position (see figure 7.15a). As usual, ensure you use your abdominal muscles rather than your arms to generate momentum. Lift your upper body so that your shoulder blades leave the floor (see figure 7.15b). Relax your neck muscles by picking a point on the ceiling to look at.

Imagine compressing and releasing a spring as you sit up and lower yourself down.

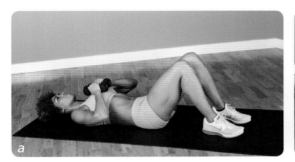 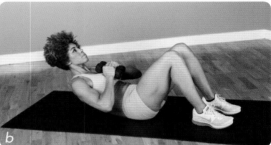

Figure 7.15   Resisted sit-up.

ARM BLAST

Exercise Focus

Biceps and triceps

How To

Assume a sturdy stance, either with feet placed hip-width apart or in a split lunge position for extra stability. Keep one dumbbell by your side and lift the other dumbbell and place it behind your head, pointing your elbow towards the ceiling (see figure 7.16a). Now, simultaneously lift both dumbbells, performing a bicep curl with the lower arm and a triceps extension with the top arm (see figure 7.16b).

> *Ensure that the upper arms do not move on either the triceps extension or the biceps curl.*

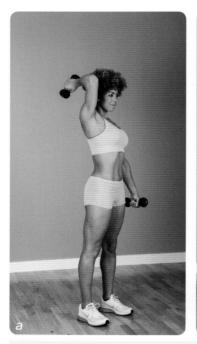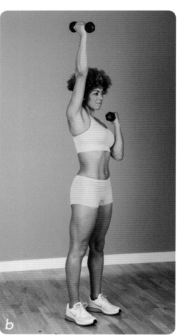

Figure 7.16   Arm blast.

RESISTED REVERSE CURL

Exercise Focus

Abdominals

How To

Lie on your back and draw your knees up to your chest, then cross your feet. Carefully secure one dumbbell between your feet. Place your hands on the floor by your side, with the palms facing upwards, so you can't use them to give extra push (see figure 7.17a). Now, relax your neck as you tighten your abdominal muscles to bring your knees closer to your chest and lift your bum off the floor (see figure 7.17b).

Avoid using your legs to kick yourself up. Work against gravity on the way down to get the most benefit for your midsection.

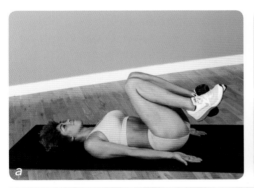 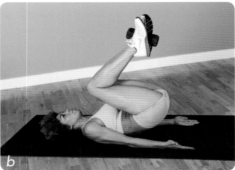

Figure 7.17   Resisted reverse curl.

Medicine Ball Exercises

Following are several medicine ball exercises that you can choose to use in your workouts.

SQUAT THROW

Exercise Focus

Glutes, quadriceps, hamstrings, deltoids and core

How To

Stand with your feet hip-width apart and facing front. Hold the ball down in front of your body with slightly bent arms. Slowly squat down until your thighs are parallel with the floor, lowering the ball between your legs (see figure 7.18a). Keep your shoulders back and your abdominal muscles pulled in and, pressing your heels into the ground, use your legs to explode up. At the same time, swing and throw the ball as high as possible directly upwards (see figure 7.18b). It should land on the ground just in front of you.

For obvious reasons, this is best suited to a sports hall, high-ceiling gym or outdoor setting.

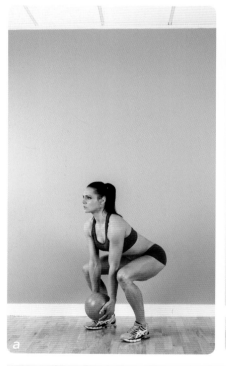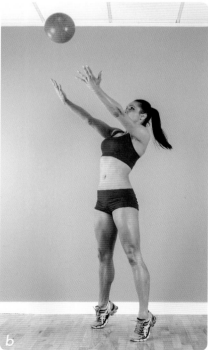

Figure 7.18   Squat throw.

CHOP

Exercise Focus

Obliques

How To

Stand with your feet a little wider than hip-width apart. Hold the ball in both hands and position it behind and above your left ear (see figure 7.19a). Bear your weight on the ball of your right foot, with the heel raised, not flat. Keeping your arms extended, move the ball diagonally down and across the body. Hinge at your hip so you end with the ball near your right knee or foot (see figure 7.19b). Return to the start position by reversing the same pattern.

Keep your abdominal muscles engaged throughout and rotate your left leg or foot in as you chop down.

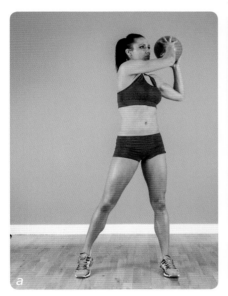 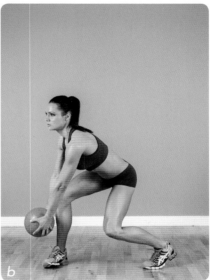

Figure 7.19   Chop.

SPRINT PASS

Exercise Focus

Glutes, quadriceps, hamstrings, pectorals, triceps and core

How To

Assume a crouched, sprinter's start position and place both hands on the ball that is resting on the floor, just in front of you (see figure 7.20a). As you explode up, pick the ball up to chest level (see figure 7.20b) and throw it straight out in front of you to a partner or at a wall, as far and fast as you can (see figure 7.20c). At the same time, drive through with your rear leg so that you actually sprint forward a couple of steps. Alternate the lead leg on each repetition.

Concentrate on your co-ordination and aim for a simultaneous movement of the legs and arms, rather than stand then throw then run.

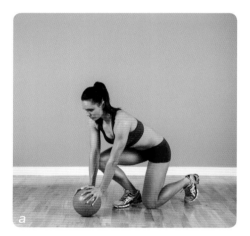

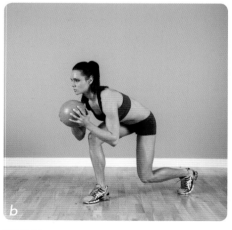

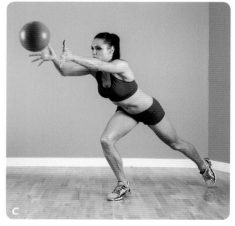

Figure 7.20   Sprint pass.

V SIT-UP

Exercise Focus

Abdominals

How To

Lie on your back, with feet lifted to the ceiling and knees bent, holding the ball above and behind your head in both hands, so that it is also resting on the floor (see figure 7.21a). Strongly contract the abdominal muscles to raise your shoulders off the floor, bringing the ball over and in front of you with the arms extended, reaching the ball to your feet (see figure 7.21b).

Avoid swinging the ball to generate momentum. Try to keep your head, neck and lower back in a neutral (or comfortable) position throughout the exercise.

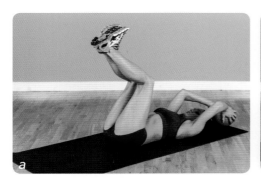
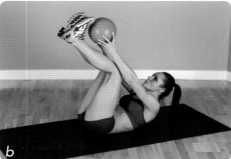

Figure 7.21   V sit-up.

PRESS-UP

Exercise Focus

Pectorals, deltoids and triceps

How To

Start in the press-up position, with your hands slightly wider than shoulder-width apart and one hand on the ball. You can assume the full press-up position or modify it by placing your knees on the floor (see figure 7.22a). To ensure your lower spine maintains its natural curve, do not drop your hips down. Lower the chest close to the floor by bending the elbows out to the side, concentrating on alignment so that the whole body moves as one unit (see figure 7.22b). Push up to return to the start position, keeping the abdominal muscles pulled in.

Try not to twist your trunk.

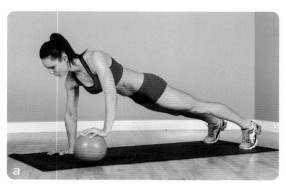 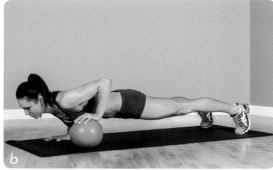

Figure 7.22   Press-up.

LUNGE

Exercise Focus

Quadriceps, hamstrings and glutes

How To

Assume a long lunge position, with your feet placed hip-width apart to give stability and with your rear foot resting on the ball (see figure 7.23a). Keeping your upper body upright, slowly lower into a lunge by bending both knees as far as is comfortable (see figure 7.23b). Strongly contract your thighs and buttocks to return up to the start position.

Balance will be a challenge, but do not twist your hips, as this will generate a torque on the knee joint that could lead to injury.

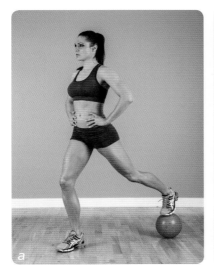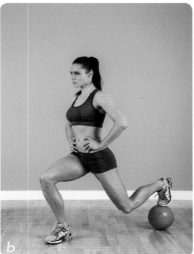

Figure 7.23   Lunge.

CHEST PRESS

Exercise Focus

Pectorals and triceps

How To

Lie on your back, with knees bent and feet flat on the floor, and hold the ball in both hands just above your chest (see figure 7.24a). Engage your core by pulling in your tummy and waist, then explosively push the ball upwards and let it fly straight up to the ceiling (see figure 7.24b). Softly catch the ball as it drops and immediately lower it to your chest, then powerfully push again.

You may need a few gentle attempts to get your technique right, as slight variation in angle of push or balance of pressure from left to right will result in losing control of the ball.

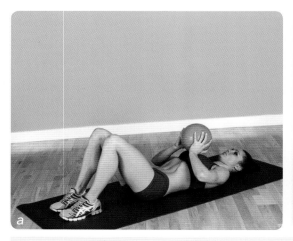
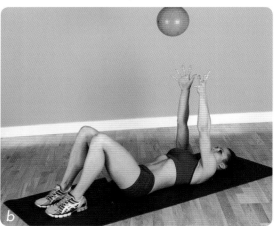

Figure 7.24   Chest press.

LEAN

Exercise Focus

Core

How To

Kneel on the floor, creating a wide base and lifting your buttocks so you are not sitting on your legs. Hold the ball in both hands and place them directly above your head but also slightly forward of the line of the body (see figure 7.25a). Keeping your navel pulled in and your hips in line, slowly hinge at the waist to lower to one side (see figure 7.25b). Move your upper body as one and maintain a long spine. You may only move a small distance, but you should target the core muscles effectively rather than letting your chest twist, as your hips will quickly follow, putting undue strain on your lower back.

You must perform this exercise slowly, with control of your momentum and with full awareness.

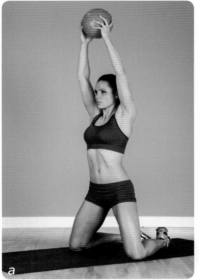 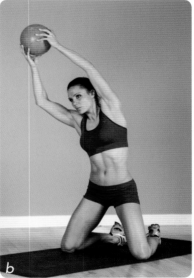

Figure 7.25   Lean.

Kettlebell Exercises

Following are several kettlebell exercises that you can choose to use in your workouts.

ALTERNATE SWING

Exercise Focus

Glutes, quadriceps, hamstrings, deltoids and core

How To

Standing with your feet slightly wider than hip-width apart, bend your knees and take the handle with one hand in an overhand grip with a slight bend in your elbow (see figure 7.26a). Hold the weight in a hanging position between the legs, but try to keep your upper body near upright, with your chest lifted and shoulder blades drawn back and down. Your free arm should be out to the side. Initiate the swing (see figure 7.26b) and rock your hips forwards rather than using your arm or shoulder to lift. Raise the kettlebell upwards with momentum and focus on a deliberate hip thrust at top of movement. Aim to lift no higher than eye level, with the kettlebell ending in a horizontal position (see figure 7.26c). As you near the end of the upward swing, bring your free arm in and swiftly swap hands at the still point, just before the kettlebell begins its descent. Allow gravity to bring it downwards, but ensure that you exert some control.

Engage your core muscles at all times by pulling in your tummy and your waist to protect your lower spine. Check that you do not round the spine at the bottom of the movement.

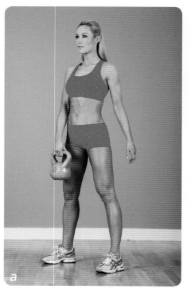
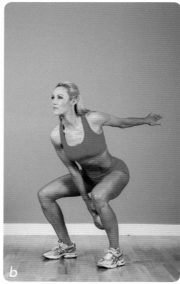
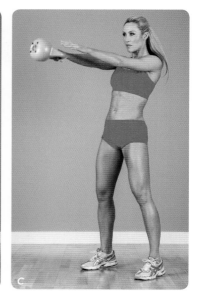

Figure 7.26   Alternate swing.

SINGLE-LEG DEAD LIFT

Exercise Focus

Hamstrings, glutes and core

How To

Standing tall with your feet together, hold the kettlebell in front of your body in both hands, with your elbows slightly bent, your shoulders pulled back and your deep abdominal muscles engaged to support your lower spine (see figure 7.27a). Hinge at your hips to lower the weight towards the ground, keeping your tummy pulled in, shoulders back and neck in a relaxed position (i.e., let your head drop) so you look to the ground about 2 metres in front of you. Aim to lower the weight until your upper body is parallel with the ground. At the same time, lift one leg up behind you, extended out straight (see figure 7.27b). Do not allow your hips to twist. Then straighten back up by driving your hips forwards.

Concentrate on keeping your back long and the top of your head as far away from your tailbone as possible.

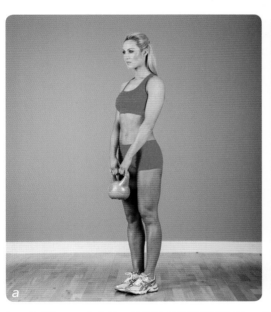 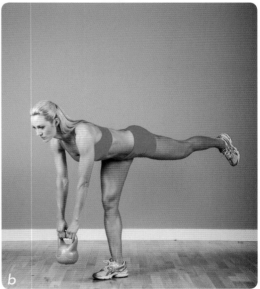

Figure 7.27   Single-leg dead lift.

LUNGE TWIST

Exercise Focus

Glutes, quadriceps, hamstrings, core and obliques

How To

Hold the kettlebell close to your body at chest height and assume a standing position, with your chest lifted and abdominal muscles pulled in tight (see figure 7.28a). Step one foot behind you with a long stride length, and bend both knees to lower yourself down into a lunge. Simultaneously turn your body as far as is comfortable to the side of your front leg, keeping the hips fixed and rotating from above the waist (see figure 7.28b). Alternate legs on the rear lunge.

Focus on generating the rotation with the deep oblique muscles in your waist rather than letting your arms take the lead.

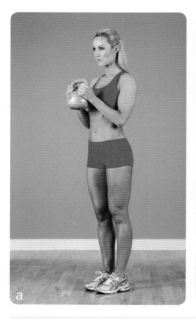 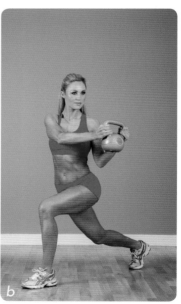

Figure 7.28   Lunge twist.

ONE-HAND PLIÉ LIFT

Exercise Focus

Glutes, quadriceps, hamstrings, adductors, deltoids and core

How To

Take your feet out wide and squat down, with your knees out, to hold the kettlebell on the floor between your legs (see figure 7.29*a*). Aim to keep your chest lifted and shoulders back rather than rounding your spine down as you pick up the weight. Keeping your core muscles strongly engaged, bend your elbow to lift the weight from the floor as you jump upwards off the ground (see figure 7.29*b*). Then flick your wrist to roll it onto the back of your hand and press the weight up overhead whilst jumping your feet in to meet in the middle as you land (see figure 7.29*c*). Then walk your feet out wide again as you swing the weight forward and lower it down to the floor.

Do not let your shoulders drop forwards when lowering the weight.

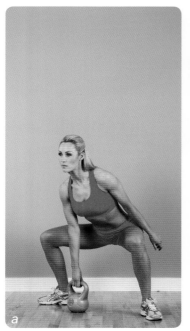 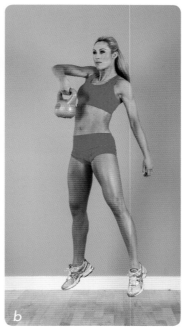 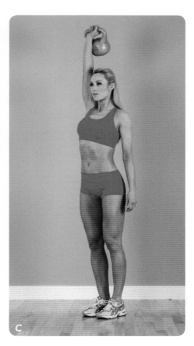

Figure 7.29   One-hand plié lift.

PRONE ROW

Exercise Focus

Upper back, biceps and core

How To

Assume either a full or modified (knees down) press-up position, with one hand on the floor and the other on the kettlebell (see figure 7.30a). Check your alignment, particularly making sure that your hips have not dropped to the floor, causing an exaggerated curve in your lower back.

Next, shift all your body weight across to your free arm, without twisting your torso and perform a row with the weight, lifting it up to your shoulder (see figure 7.30b). Slowly lower the kettlebell and reset your posture before the next lift. This is not easy, so take your time.

Keep *the movement to a minimum, and only use your arm to row.*

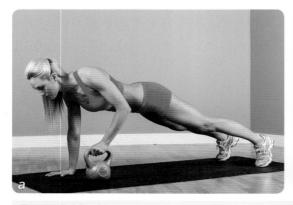 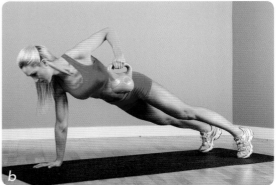

Figure 7.30   Prone row.

TURKISH STAND-UP

Exercise Focus

Glutes, quadriceps, hamstrings, deltoids and core

How To

Lie on your back, holding the kettlebell in one hand directly above your chest (see figure 7.31a). Strongly contract your abdominal muscles to lift your upper body whilst bringing one foot in close to your backside (see figure 7.31b), and then drive onto the near foot and step up into a standing position (see figure 7.31c). Now reverse this by placing one knee down first and slowly lowering until you are lying flat again. Keep your arm with the kettlebell fully extended at all times.

You may need to place your free hand on the floor for extra push as you drive onto the near foot and step up into a standing position.

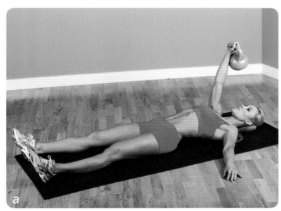

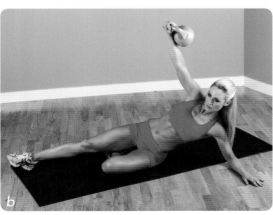

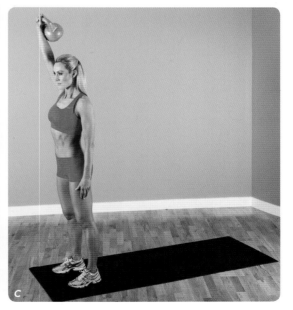

Figure 7.31 Turkish stand-up.

SINGLE-SHOULDER PRESS

Exercise Focus

Deltoids, triceps and core

How To

Stand tall, with your feet hip-width apart, knees slightly bent and postural muscles engaged. Lift the kettlebell to shoulder level, with the weight resting on the back of your wrist (see figure 7.32a). Bend your knees to drop your body weight just slightly, then press through your heels and drive from the legs. Use this momentum to initiate the shoulder press, lifting the weight up overhead (see figure 7.32b).

Be careful not to lock out the elbow.

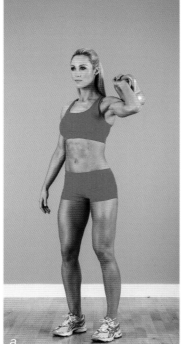 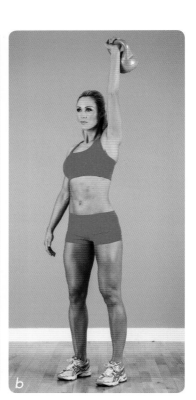

Figure 7.32   Single-shoulder press.

RUSSIAN TWIST

Exercise Focus

Core and obliques

How To

Stand with your feet hip-width apart and hold the kettlebell with both hands, keeping your elbows bent and into the body (see figure 7.33a). Contract the obliques at the side of your waist to rotate your torso and move the kettlebell to one side as far as is comfortable (see figure 7.33b). Return to the centre and repeat to the other side. You can also perform this exercise sitting on a fitness ball or on the floor. Whichever option you choose, focus on your alignment, with your navel drawn back towards your spine, chest lifted and neck long.

Try to keep your lower body stable and your hips square to the front. Remember, slower is better with this exercise.

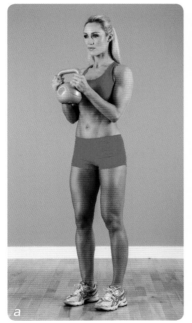 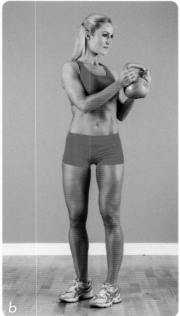

Figure 7.33   Russian twist.

Body-Weight Exercises

Please don't think we're suggesting that joining a gym or purchasing home fitness kit are worthless investments. In fact, we believe quite the opposite. They can both be vital contributing factors in helping you to stick to a regular exercise routine. Let's be honest, however, in this current age of austerity some of us are going to have to find ways to cut our financial outgoings, but the good news is that this doesn't mean you have to cut back on your workouts. Mother Nature has kindly provided us the best workout aid, completely free of charge—gravity. Using just your own body weight, we've created a range of exercises you can do to target all your problem areas and ensure you burn a truckload of calories.

HINDU PRESS-UP

Exercise Focus

Pectorals, deltoids and triceps

How To

Start in a downward dog pose, with your hands and feet on the floor, your backside lifted up towards the heavens and your tummy pulled in tight. Pull your shoulders away from your ears to lengthen your neck, and drop the top of your head toward the floor (see figure 7.34*a*). Now bend your elbows and take your chin close to the floor, shifting your body weight forwards so your chin traces a path close to the floor, between your hands (see figure 7.34*b*). Next, extend through your back to lift your face up and forwards (see figure 7.34*c*), then return to the start position. You will perform three movements here—shifting down and forwards, lifting up and then returning up and back to the start—but you should aim to link them together in one smooth movement.

Keep your chin as close to the floor as possible as you shift your weight forwards.

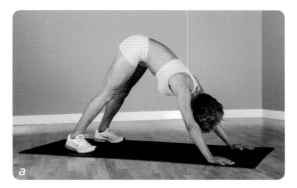

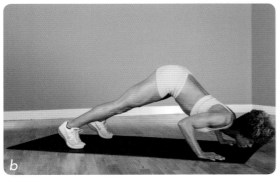
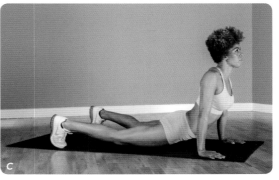

Figure 7.34   Hindu press-up.

SINGLE-LEG BRIDGE

Exercise Focus

Hamstrings, glutes and core

How To

Lie on your back with one leg extended and the other bent at the knee so your foot is flat on the floor (see figure 7.35a). Take a moment to locate your neutral spine by gently tipping your lower pelvis up and down until you find the position that feels most comfortable for your lower back. This will gently curve your lumbar spine away from the floor. Begin by engaging your core muscles—drawing up your pelvic floor, pulling in your navel and squeezing your oblique muscles in the waist. This will brace your lumbo-pelvic region so that your lower spine remains in the neutral position when you move, protecting it from potential injury.

> *Keep your body in a long line and your core engaged so that your hips do not sag or arch upwards.*

Now use a strong contraction in the buttocks and hamstring muscles to press the planted foot into the ground and lift your lower body off the floor (see figure 7.35b). Avoid placing stress on the top part of your spine, shoulders or neck.

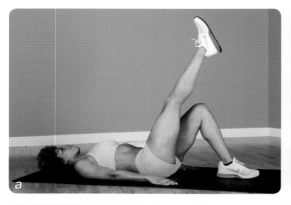 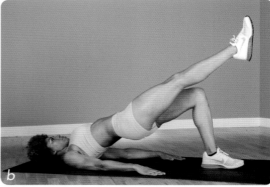

Figure 7.35   Single-leg bridge.

SPLIT LUNGE

Exercise Focus

Glutes, quadriceps, hamstrings and core

Equipment

Step, platform, chair

How To

Stand a long stride length in front of a step, platform or chair, facing away from it. Raise one leg and reach it behind you to rest the ball of the foot on the prop (see figure 7.36a). Point the rear foot down rather than out, and place it so that the feet are not in line, but are hip-width apart to assist balance. Bend the knee on your front standing leg to lower your body down, taking the rear knee directly down towards the floor (see figure 7.36b). Take care not to twist this rear knee. Go as low as you comfortably can and then contract through your thighs and buttocks to lift yourself back to the starting position, keeping your tummy pulled in tight and your head up throughout the movement.

If your front knee bends beyond your supporting foot at the bottom of the lunge, lengthen your stride position.

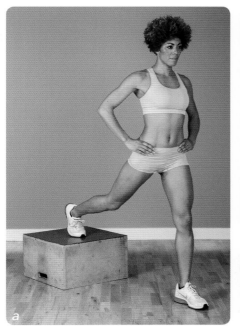 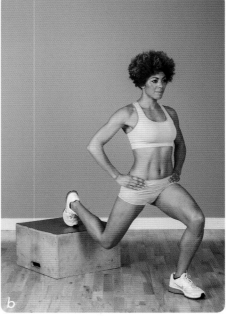

Figure 7.36 Split lunge.

TRICEPS PRESS

Exercise Focus

Triceps and obliques

How To

Lie on the floor on your side with knees bent and your top hand placed flat on the floor directly in front of your chest (see figure 7.37a). Press the hand into the floor and extend your arm to lift your torso off the ground, as high as you can (see figure 7.37b), then slowly return to the start position. Keep your core muscles engaged, pulling in the navel and waist and lifting up the pelvic floor to keep your torso rigid.

> *Resist the temptation to twist your body as you lift or to use the oblique muscles in the waist. Let the arm do all the work.*

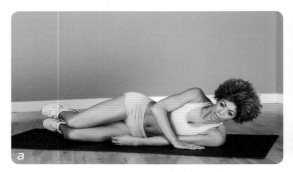 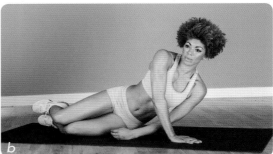

Figure 7.37   Triceps press.

SINGLE-LEG CALF RAISE

Exercise Focus

Calves and core

Equipment

Step or stair

How To

Stand on one leg on a step platform or the bottom step of a flight of stairs, holding a handrail or using the wall for balance. Place your foot right on the front of the step so that your heel hangs over the edge (see figure 7.38a). Roll onto the ball of your foot, lifting your heel as high as possible through a strong contraction in your calf muscles (see figure 7.38b). Then lower yourself down gently and drop your heel below the level of the step, working through your full comfortable range of motion. Throughout the exercise, ensure the knee on your standing leg is not locked out, but is slightly soft.

If your balance will allow, you could try the exercise without holding on for support, as this will introduce extra benefit for your core muscles.

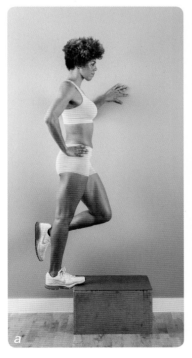 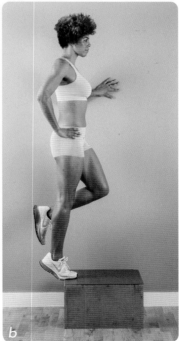

Figure 7.38   Single-leg calf raise.

SIDE LUNGE

Exercise Focus

Quadriceps, hamstrings, glutes and core

How To

Start by standing with your feet together and your weight evenly balanced. Now take a wide step out to the left side with your left leg, placing your foot so that it points slightly outwards in the direction you are stepping. In a smooth, continuous movement, bend your left knee, keeping your right leg straight and simultaneously hinging at the hip to reach your hands towards the ground (see figure 7.39).

Focus on your alignment. The hinge at the hip is not a rounding of your spine, so keep your core engaged at all times and your shoulder blades drawn back and down, away from your ears.

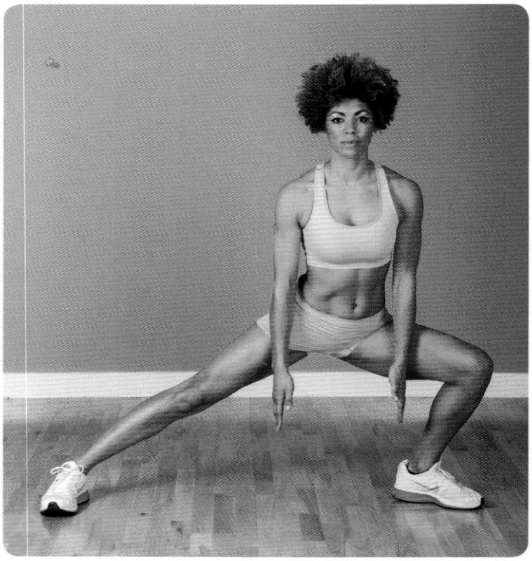

Next, drive through your left foot to push back to the start position. Complete the target number of repetitions before changing sides; do not alternate.

Figure 7.39   Side lunge.

PLANK LIFT

Exercise Focus

Core, deltoids, glutes and triceps

How To

Assume a plank position, with your hands directly under your shoulders and your lower back in a comfortable place (see figure 7.40*a*). Do not allow your hips to sag towards the floor or your bum to stick up in the air. Now focus on your centre, really pulling in at the navel and the waist and up from your pelvic floor to fix your hips in space. Without moving anything else, slowly lift one leg. Hold it steady and then lift the opposite arm out to the side (see figure 7.40*b*). The aim is to challenge your core muscles to hold your body in position, without twisting or dropping your hips.

This is a tough exercise, so you might need to start with just a leg lift for a while. Progress to the full lift when you feel stronger.

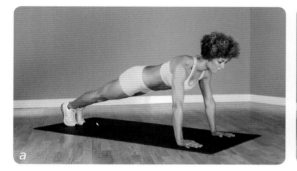 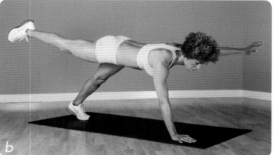

Figure 7.40   Plank lift.

CRUNCH

Exercise Focus

Abdominals

How To

Lie on your back with knees bent so your feet are flat on the floor, and rest your hands on your thighs (see figure 7.41a). Tightly tense your upper abdominal muscles to lift your shoulders off the floor, reaching your hands forwards. At the same time, strongly contract the lower abdominal muscles to lift your feet off the floor (see figure 7.41b). Return to the start position, lowering yourself down slowly and working against rather than with gravity. For additional benefit, try to hold the raised position for a couple of seconds before descending again.

If you begin to feel stress in your neck muscles, place one hand behind your head for support and simply reach with the other hand as you lift up.

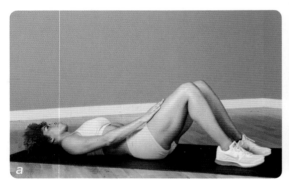
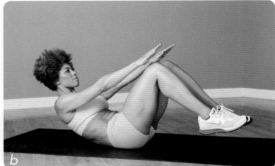

Figure 7.41   Crunch.

RESISTANCE TRAINING WORKOUT FORMATS

Whatever your favoured choice of resistance, it is advisable to vary your workouts to avoid the plateau effect, whereby your body becomes accustomed to your routine and so responds poorly, slowing down your progress.

Before introducing specific workout formats, let's take a moment to demystify a current hot topic in the fitness domain—functional training. Although much has been said and written, unfortunately, not all of it has been helpful. A functional exercise can be described as one that improves specific strength that will then influence sports performance or everyday tasks. To illustrate this, take the examples of a jump athlete who needs to develop explosive strength in her take-off leg and a woman who needs to be able to walk up a flight of stairs carrying a baby. The former might practice single-leg squats at speed, whilst the new mum would benefit from holding a weight in her hands and performing step-ups onto a platform. The converse of these is an exercise that is purely designed to achieve aesthetic benefits, such as a traditional sit-up, a movement we only use twice a day, when we get out of bed in the morning and then return at night. The vital difference is that functional exercises train the movement, whilst aesthetic (body-building) training targets the muscle. A sensible approach would be to include a mix of exercises, so promoting improvements in both domains.

The following four formats can be applied to the resistance machine and free-weights routines.

Pyramids

This gym format works on varying the resistance and therefore the number of repetitions on each set for all exercises. It can be tweaked either as an ascending (resistance from light to heavy repetitions from high to low), descending (resistance from heavy to light repetitions from low to high), or full pyramid (combines both to go from light to heavy and then back to light load, with repetitions decreasing and then increasing again). A rest of about 2 minutes between each set is usual. Pyramids are useful for improving both strength and endurance as you work through a varying repetition range, targeting both the slow- and fast-twitch fibres. Be warned that this is not easy, as each set must be performed to failure. The intensity is high. In addition, if you take this approach to every exercise or routine, you will need plenty of time.

(continued)

(continued)

Pre-Exhaust Sets

The theory here is based on the fact that often, when working the larger muscle groups, it's the smaller ones assisting that fatigue first, so you don't get to the point of momentary muscular fatigue that is required to stimulate the adaptive responses that lead to stronger muscles. The answer, then, is to perform a set of isolation exercises (using just one muscle group) before performing a compound exercise (requiring several muscles to work together).

Negative Training

When a weight is lifted, either directly (as in the case of a dumbbell and barbell) or indirectly (as with the plates on a fixed-weight machine), it should be lowered with some resistance to ensure gravity doesn't send it crashing back down. This is referred to as the negative phase of the exercise. Negatives describe just performing this second part of the lifting exercise, with a partner assisting you on the lift of the weight. The beauty of this approach is that it allows you to work with loads that are greater than your maximum lift, leading to considerable strength improvements and the psychological gain of handling larger weights that can in turn promote greater volumes of training in future. There is a possible disadvantage of this technique, however, as research suggests it is linked with more pronounced muscle soreness on the day following your workout.

Drop Sets

This is actually a modified version of the descending pyramid, the difference being that very little (or no!) rest is taken between each set. The easiest route to achieving this is on fixed-weight machines, as you can very quickly pull the pin out of the weight stack and place it in a lighter position. The usual target is performing an additional three sets after the initial set to failure. Since these should also be performed to total fatigue, this is not for the faint-hearted. The first set you will perform is at a heavy load, so you must warm up thoroughly beforehand. The advantage of this method is that you can achieve complete overload of the target muscle groups in a fairly short space of time. One complete round of descending sets is enough.

Peripheral Heart Action (PHA)

The PHA approach is most commonly applied to circuit training sessions. It allows for a high volume of exercise in minimum time. This versatile format can be used with all the resistance modes previously described.

By alternating exercises between the upper and lower body, one muscle group has the opportunity to rest while another is exerting, so specific rests are not required. The cardiovascular system also benefits, as it is called on to constantly shift blood from one area of the body to another location. This vascular shunt, as it is known, is brought about by the muscles' demand for oxygen when they are working. This leads to a greater total calorie burn for the workout.

AT A GLANCE

- Muscles are made up of two different fibre types: fast-twitch and slow-twitch.
- Strength training aids weight-loss efforts.
- For pure strength gains, you need to lift heavy weights for only around 5 repetitions.
- More commonly, though, the target is 12 repetitions, which produces improvements in strength and also endurance.
- In both cases, however, it's crucial to work with loads that are heavy enough to result in fatigue on the last couple of repetitions of each set.
- As you get stronger, you must increase the resistance or your visible results will stall.
- Ideally, your routine should incorporate both functional exercises that train movements and aesthetic exercises that train muscles.

8

Power Up

What comes to mind when you think about being powerful? Which sports, athletes and physiques do you visualise? Most people associate power with competitive sport and professional athletes, but the truth is that we all require power for everyday life. It is vital for many functional demands and movements, such as sport, play and active daily living (mowing the lawn and climbing a flight of stairs), and also during emergencies, such as preventing a fall or dodging an obstacle. Consequently, increasing power will increase your efficiency and ability to do all tasks, as well as enhance sporting performance. In a primal world where danger lurked around every corner, our ability to move fast determined our survival. In fact, we were designed to move quickly, originally to avoid a charging herd of mastodons or to run down small game for dinner! Primal needs aside, power training has an incredible ability to improve your physique and help you lose weight whilst spending much less time exercising than you would with a typical steady state cardio workout.

POWER DEVELOPMENT

Quite simply, power is defined as strength expressed at high speed. For example, a conventional squat with additional weight is an example of strength, whereas a squat performed explosively (for example, as a squat jump) is power. Most movements performed at speed, such as sprinting, are power moves. Developing muscular power to enhance these movements is different from developing muscular strength and endurance.

To take this further, understand that strength is independent of time. That is, it is simply the maximal force a muscle (or group of muscles) can exert. Power, however, is an expression of how quickly that force can be generated, for example, when accelerating, jumping or throwing. Here are a few benefits of including power workouts and exercises into your training plan:

- *Time efficiency*—A power-based workout (sprints or jumps) cannot be sustained effectively for a long period of time. In fact, it's unlikely you will perform any one exercise for longer than 30 seconds before your power declines. For most people, 10 seconds is enough to begin with. Consequently, only short sets and reps are required to achieve a fatigued state and elicit performance gains.

- *Muscle tone and definition*—A higher percentage of your muscle fibres are recruited when you work quickly and explosively. More muscle-fibre activation equals more complete muscular definition. Visualise the lean, toned body of a high jumper or beach volleyball player; they are some of the most powerful yet most aesthetically pleasing athletes and they do lots of power training!

- *Fat burning*—Power exercises have a high energy demand; therefore, they increase your metabolism and burn fat faster than high-volume workouts performed slowly. They also suppress your appetite due to elevated body temperature in the hours following exercise, as well as develop more calorie-burning lean muscle and improve insulin sensitivity (highly worked muscles learn not only to burn glucose effectively but also to absorb glucose, transported by insulin, after workouts).

- *Anti-ageing and well-being*—Maximal explosive efforts minimise the effects of ageing by promoting the release of testosterone, human growth hormone and serotonin, which are beneficial for women as well as men. These endocrine responses help promote balance in the autonomic nervous system and benefit the processes of growth, recovery and regeneration, all of which create an environment for positive change.

- *Improved sports performance*—As already stated, most sports rely on power at some stage. The more you work to increase both your absolute power and power endurance (see following sections), the better your sporting performance will be.

- *Improved daily activity performance*—The more reactive your muscles become, the faster they will respond to stimuli and will ensure you can go about your daily activities more efficiently and with minimal stress. This can apply to tasks as simple as walking up a hill or moving furniture.

- *Fun and focused mind*—There's not a chance of becoming bored during a power workout! Your body and mind are invigorated. Concentration remains high and results occur fast. Progression is easily measured through timed runs, jump heights and throw distance to ensure you remain driven by goals and results.

WEIGHT-LOSS TIP   Power training can be a great calorie burner, as it involves the recruitment of a large number of muscle fibres. As more muscle fibres become active and, subsequently adapt and develop, the faster your metabolic rate will be.

POWER AND PLYOMETRICS

You may have heard the word *plyometrics* being thrown around by athletes, coaches and others in the know. Plyometrics are extremely effective exercises for producing power, and they are often used by women to improve sports performance. They are essentially a series of explosive exercises that stretch your muscles like a rubber band and then contract them again quickly, enabling you to produce fast, powerful movements. Plyometrics actually reduce the time it takes for a muscle in the human body to contract, which means that the muscle can exert a greater amount of power and force.

Most sports—athletics (sprinting, throwing and jumping), cycling, netball, football, basketball and swimming—include plyometric power movements. Even the serene nature of a yoga class can involve some power moves such as when you leap out of a downward dog position into a standing forward bend or kick up into a headstand. Many fitness classes familiar to you feature power components, including spinning, circuits and kettlebell workouts, to mention just a few.

So why not utilize the elasticity of your muscles and benefit from plyometrics in your workout? Typical plyometric exercises include jumps and bounding. Our favourites are detailed later in this chapter.

POWER TRAINING METHODS AND EXERCISES

We all have individual needs when it comes to working out, and the same is true of selecting the right type of power training for you. For example, some athletes train to be able to perform one maximal explosive action. Examples include a weightlifter, shot-putter, long-jumper and javelin thrower. These athletes need to train for pure or explosive power. Some athletes are required to complete these controlled explosive moves repeatedly but continuously for a short period of time. This applies to sprinters, who need to train for short-term power. Other athletes will need to perform repeated power moves, taking very little recovery between efforts. They need to deliver fast and at short notice, often in response to an external stimulus. This is typical for boxers and for volleyball, tennis and netball players, and they need not only pure power, but power endurance, which develops the anaerobic lactic-acid buffering system described in chapter 6: Go Anaerobic. One or all of these may apply to you for your own sport, activity or lifestyle requirements, so we want to make sure you know how to train specifically for the type of power that you need. We also want to make this fun and varied, and in keeping with any other special requirements you may have.

POWER TRAINING SAFETY AND CONSIDERATIONS

Due to the high-impact nature of most power exercises, you must consider some prerequisites and put safety measures in place:

- Condition your body before attempting any power workout. You need good joint stability and muscle strength, as well as good technique and flexibility, to prevent injury and ensure you get the most from your power workout. For example, it is no use performing squat jumps until you have established a good movement pattern for a conventional squat, based on achieving full range with good posture and with sufficient load. Adding a jump increases the stress on your joints as the force factor increases, magnifying any movement imbalances.

- Warm up with some light cardio and muscle activation through drills that replicate the movements you are to perform before doing any full explosive actions (see chapter 4: Warming Up and Cooling Down for examples and details).

- For an explosive power workout, ensure you are in a rested state, with no fatigue lingering from earlier workouts or exercises. Perform the exercises at the beginning of your workout for best results and to avoid injury from fatigue. For a power endurance workout, select greater repetition numbers with shorter rest but do exercises requiring less impact and risk than those selected for explosive power.

- Progress sensibly—When you first start power training, opt for a shorter exercise time and lower-impact exercises, such as cycling or sprinting up a steep hill and then walking down again for repeat efforts. Progress gradually based on adaptation and mastery of each movement pattern.

- Ideally, you should perform power workouts only when your motivation is high. Half-hearted attempts can result in poor performance and injury.

- Expect DOMS (delayed-onset muscle soreness) after a power workout, especially if you are trying something new or stepping up your workout level. This is due to the stress response to the body that occurs—hormone levels, muscular breakdown and joint inflammation. Consider good post-workout nutrition, supplements and treatments such as massage (see chapter 3: Nutrition Matters and chapter 4: Warming Up and Cooling Down). However, you can expect to quickly adapt to a power workout routine.

- Clear the area you will be exercising in of bags, equipment and other objects that you do not want to land or step on during the movement.

- Ideally, you should work with a partner or trainer who can observe your technique and instruct on whether you are landing safely and executing the movement correctly.

This section describes the exercise methods you can use to increase your power as well as the most effective exercises for each. These methods include the use of body-weight exercises, plyometrics, sprints and equipment-based exercises. We have outlined the necessary points to help you understand their purpose. For details of full workouts incorporating these exercises, check out chapter 11: Sample Workouts and Programmes.

WEIGHT-LOSS TIP

If your goal is weight loss, steer yourself towards the power endurance exercises to blast more calories compared with single power explosive exercises.

Body-Weight Plyometric Exercises

Body-weight plyometric exercises for power are perfect for general conditioning, as an introduction to power training and for sports requiring all over power endurance (football, volleyball, netball, boxing), especially when performed as a circuit. These exercises are time saving and work your whole body.

BURPEES

Exercise Focus
Total-body explosive power

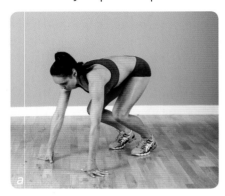

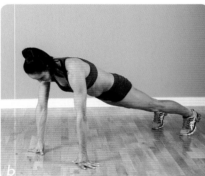

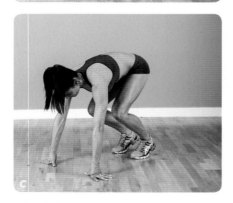

How To
Stand with your feet together, and then bend at your knees, lean forwards and place your hands flat on the floor just in front of your feet (see figure 8.1*a*). Jump both feet backwards to create a straight-arm plank position (see figure 8.1*b*) before jumping your feet back again towards your hands (see figure 8.1*c*), performing a squat thrust. Finally jump upwards from this squatting position, driving your legs straight and arms behind you (see figure 8.1*d*). Land and repeat.

Aim for maximum height on the jump, and keep all phases of the movement continuous.

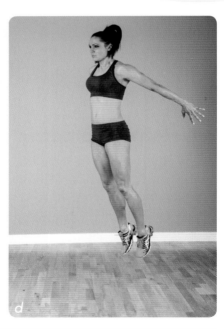

Figure 8.1   Burpees.

WIDE-TO-NARROW SQUAT JUMPS

Exercise Focus

Power exercise for adductors, quadriceps and glutes

How To

Start in a wide squat position, with the toes and knees facing outwards (see figure 8.2a). Bend at the knees and jump upwards (see figure 8.2b), bringing your feet together as you do so. Land with both feet together (see figure 8.2c), and then immediately jump back to the wide squat position to repeat the movement.

Aim for maximal height with each jump and for good depth in each squat position.

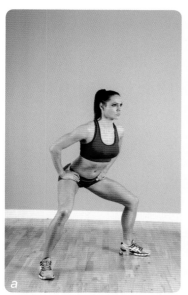
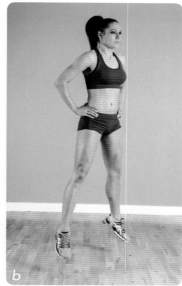
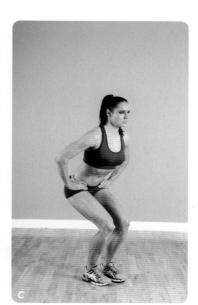

Figure 8.2   Wide-to-narrow squat jumps.

MOUNTAIN CLIMBERS

Exercise Focus

Knee drive for power endurance

How To

Start in a straight-arm plank position with your feet shoulder-width apart and your bottom slightly raised so that your body creates a V-shape. In a continuous movement, drive one knee forwards toward your chest (see figure 8.3a). Bring it immediately back again and drive the other knee forwards, as if you were sprinting (see figure 8.3b). Continue this pattern with alternating leg movements. Aim to create a near-straight position with your back leg to create as much range as possible between the knee tuck and knee drive. Keep your hips as low as your body will allow.

To allow more space to drive your knees forwards, place your hands on a raised block or step.

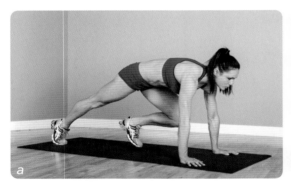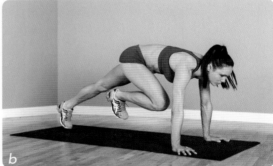

Figure 8.3   Mountain climbers.

DOUBLE-LEG CALF BOUNCES

Exercise Focus

Lower leg explosive power and ground reaction training

How To

Stand with your feet together and your hands on your hips, soften your knees and shift your weight onto the balls of your feet (see figure 8.4a). Perform small double-leg bounces with your feet in a dorsiflexed position on the upward phase (see figure 8.4b). Activate the jump with your calf muscles each time you land. To do this, keep your knees soft, but do not bend them to squat. Aim for maximal height and minimal ground contact time. For more foot muscle activation, consider performing barefoot.

To minimise impact and stress on the joints, perform on a soft mat or flat grass surface.

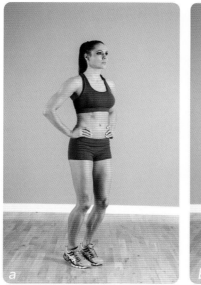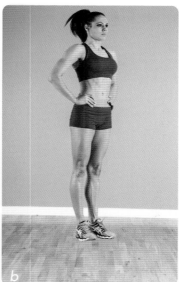

Figure 8.4   Double-leg calf bounces.

ALTERNATING SPLIT-SQUAT JUMPS

Exercise Focus

Explosive power for quadriceps and glutes

How To

Start in a split-squat position (shallow lunge position), with both feet facing forwards (see figure 8.5a). Bend both knees and drive upwards off the ground switching feet in the air (see figure 8.5b) and land with the opposite leg facing forwards (see figure 8.5c). Immediately repeat the movement, switching your legs with each repetition. Aim for height with every jump and try to land in the same spot you jumped from, rather than travelling forwards, to ensure that both your legs are working to apply equal force. You can use your arms to assist the movement and land firmly and safely. To assist your balance throughout this exercise, ensure your feet are about hip-width apart rather than in a straight line with each other.

To minimise impact and protect your joints, you can perform with your front leg on a step or box.

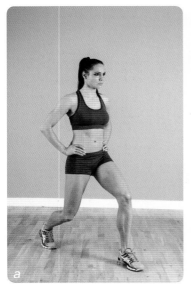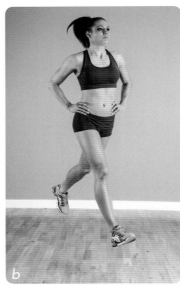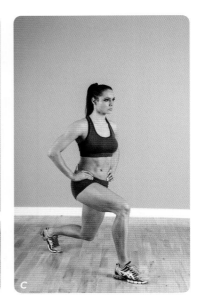

Figure 8.5   Alternating split-squat jumps.

POWER TRAINING PROTOCOL

Due to the intense and challenging nature of power training, you should incorporate it into your training programme appropriately to maximise the benefits, achieve optimal results and avoid overtraining and injury. The frequency of your power training will depend on the type of power training you are performing, your conditioning level, current training methods and sporting or activity goals, as follows.

Competitive Athletes

Perform an absolute or pure power workout one or two times per week in the 6- to 8-week phase leading up to your competitive season. During the competition season itself, your exercise intensity will naturally increase as a result of performing in your event so you can drop the specific power training frequency down to a single session per week. During your general conditioning training phases (off-season), incorporate power endurance workouts with the circuit training suggestions previously mentioned once per week.

Fitness Enthusiasts

You can incorporate power endurance exercises into your training all year round, with one or two sessions per week to gain outstanding fitness benefits and break out of any chronic cardio ruts that may have lasted for years. Once you have a good level of conditioning, add the pure power exercises. Remember to first learn the skill in its component parts and then build the intensity as you become familiar with each movement pattern. This is particularly important for Olympic lifts and bounding exercises. You can then include these pure power exercises once every 7 to 10 days. As a general rule, perform power training on the days where your energy levels and motivation are high. You should never push your body through an intense workout if you have any symptoms of fatigue, soreness, compromised immune system or another malaise.

Bounding Plyometric Exercises

These exercises improve pure explosive power. They are typically performed by women with a high level of conditioning, such as sprinters, jumpers and throwers, or by sportswomen whose sports incorporate these bounding movements. However, whether you're a competitive athlete or general exercise enthusiast, these exercises can take your workout to another level, adding dynamism and energy to your programme. If you want to look like a toned and honed athlete, then you, too, can work towards training like one.

The exercises have a high level of impact and will require some technical training in movement patterns. We suggest you begin by breaking the movements down into their component parts. Next, perform the sequence at about 60 percent maximal effort to allow your muscles, joints and neurological system to adapt over the first couple of sessions.

You will need a flat surface (a synthetic athletic track is ideal) and a 30- to 50-metre distance to work along.

ALTERNATING BOUNDS

Exercise Focus

Leg explosive power and strength and stability of landing

How To

From a start marker, move your weight onto your front leg for a stationary or rolling start (see figure 8.6a), and push off your back leg driving your front knee forwards so that this leg is parallel to the ground as you lunge forwards (see figure 8.6b). Land on the opposite leg, and then immediately drive the other leg forwards to produce a continuous succession of bounds, alternating from one leg to the other. Aim for minimal contact time with the ground (action–reaction) and try to cover as much horizontal distance as possible with each bound. Keep your hips tall and facing forwards. All joints (ankles, knees and hips) must remain strong, as any sinking as you land will minimise the effect of the stretch-shortening cycle, or elasticity effect, and will reduce power and effectiveness.

> *To stay tall, imagine that you have a piece of string attached to the top of your head and that you are being pulled upright as you move along.*

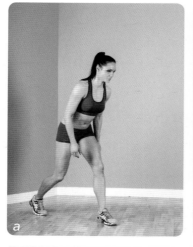 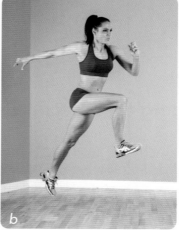

Figure 8.6 Alternating bounds.

DOUBLE-LEG BUNNY HOPS

Exercise Focus

Quadriceps power

How To

Stand with your feet shoulder-width apart, bend at the ankles, knees and hips, and bring both arms back behind you (see figure 8.7a). Explode upwards and forwards from your legs and hips, and move your arms overhead in one continuous movement (see figure 8.7b). Land with your knees and arms back down in the start position, and repeat.

The most advanced can perform these hops continuously, whilst those new to this exercise can pause to stand up and reset between hops. The secret to a good bunny hop is the smooth sequence of drive and extension from the ankles to knees to hips and arms.

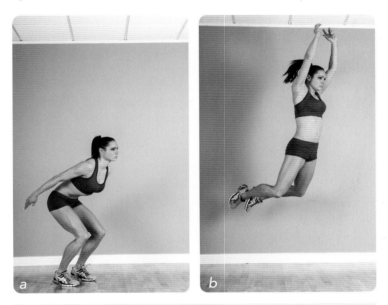

Figure 8.7   Double-leg bunny hops.

Box-Jump Plyometric Exercises

These are traditional plyometric exercises whose purpose is often to develop pure explosive power. As with bounding, these are often performed by sprinters, throwers, jumpers and weightlifters. Performing these drills requires co-ordination and practice.

The level of impact associated with each exercise depends on whether you're jumping onto a box (reduced impact) or off a box (greater impact). Therefore, select exercises carefully for your training status and requirements. Secure boxes, steps or platforms of varying heights on a clear, flat surface.

DEPTH JUMP

Exercise Focus

Lower body reactive power

Equipment

A secure box or step at approximately shin to knee height

How To

Standing in front of the box, bend at your ankles, knees and hips and bring your arms behind your body (see figure 8.8a). Jump up high bringing your arms in front of your body to assist the movement (see figure 8.8b) and land onto the box with bent knees and both feet flat (see figure 8.8c). Step back down carefully and repeat.

Beginners can use a lower box, whilst those more advanced can continue to raise the height of the box. Progress to single-leg jumps: First, try taking off from two feet and landing on one foot. Then try both taking off and landing with one foot. We advise you lower the box height when you first attempt single-leg jumps.

Aim to fully extend your body on the jump before you tuck your legs to land on the box. This will make for a better jump height and prevent you falling backwards.

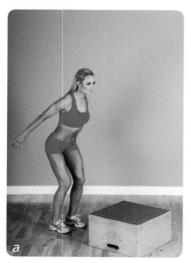
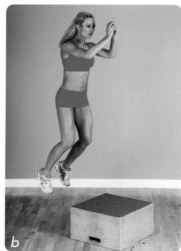
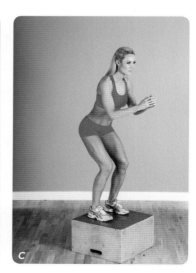

Figure 8.8   Depth jump.

VERTICAL DEPTH JUMP

Exercise Focus

Lower body reactive and explosive power

Equipment

A secure box or step at approximately knee to thigh height

How To

Stand on the front edge of the box with a clear space on the floor in front of you and lift one leg off the box and slightly in front of your body (see figure 8.9*a*). Lean forwards and step off the box, landing on both feet with your knees slightly bent and weight on the balls of your feet (see figure 8.9*b*). Immediately, jump upwards as quickly as possible, aiming for maximal height (see figure 8.9*c*). Step back up onto the box and repeat. Progress by increasing the height of your marker (see following tip) and the box.

Place a vertical jump flag or equivalent marker overhead and aim to reach up and touch it with every jump.

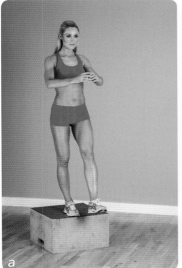
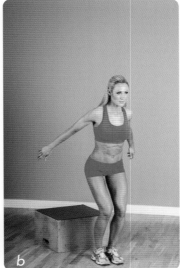
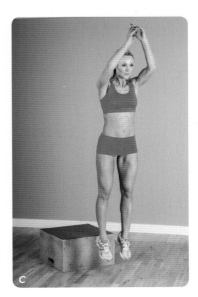

Figure 8.9 Vertical depth jump.

Medicine Ball Power Exercises

Medicine ball power exercises are perfect for general total-body conditioning and as an introduction to power training. They are also suitable for sports and activities that require all-over power endurance (football, volleyball, netball and boxing).

For each exercise, select a medicine ball of a suitable weight. You may find that you need to change weights to suit different exercises. You also need to work in a clear area, with access to a partner or a wall. When performed as a circuit, these exercises are great for calorie burning.

SEATED OVERHEAD THROW

Exercise Focus

Upper body explosive power

Equipment

2- to 5-kilogram medicine ball; wall or partner

How To

Sit on the floor with your legs straight in front of you, positioned at a throwing distance away from a wall (or partner). Raise the medicine ball above and behind your head with your arms bent (see figure 8.10a). Forcefully throw the medicine ball at the wall (or your partner) just above head height by extending at your elbows (see figure 8.10b). As the ball comes back at you, catch it with both hands. Allow the ball to recoil behind you and immediately throw it back in. Repeat back and forth. Start slowly, and gradually increase the speed throughout the repetitions. Progress to a single-handed throw with a lighter ball for added shoulder stability and precision work.

Extend and flick with your fingertips as your release the ball for efficient follow through. Keep your core strong and your chest up as you catch and recoil the ball to avoid any force absorption.

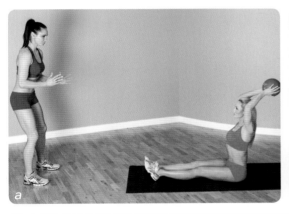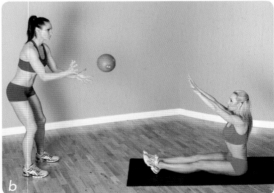

Figure 8.10   Seated overhead throw.

TANTRUM THROWS

Exercise Focus

Upper body explosive power

Equipment

2- to 5-kilogram medicine ball

How To

Stand with your feet slightly wider than shoulder-width apart and raise the medicine ball directly above your head (see figure 8.11*a*). With one continuous movement, push the ball downwards and into the ground in front of your feet, by first bending then extending your elbows and finally flicking the ball with your fingertips (see figure 8.11*b*). As the ball rebounds upwards, catch it and repeat the process. Make sure you move your head backwards as the ball rebounds so it doesn't hit you in the chin! The closer the ball lands to your feet, the more accurately it will rebound, so you won't have to move around to recover it.

You can keep your legs straight for isolated triceps activation or bend your knees as you throw for a total-body contribution.

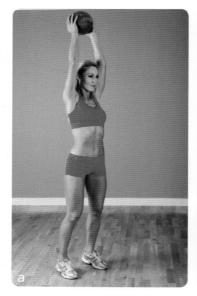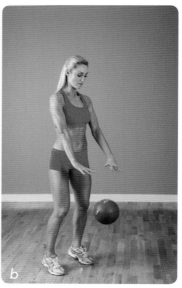

Figure 8.11   Tantrum throws.

SEATED SIDE TWIST AND THROW

Exercise Focus

Core explosive power

Equipment

2- to 5-kilogram medicine ball; wall or partner

How To

Sit on the floor perpendicular to a wall (or partner) and throwing distance away (approximately 2 metres) and with your legs stretched out in front of you and knees slightly bent. Hold the medicine ball with both hands and rotate your torso away from the wall or your partner so it's just behind your far hip (see figure 8.12a). Throw the ball at the wall or your partner by rotating your torso back in the other direction and extending your arms across your body to release the ball from shoulder height (see figure 8.12b). Receive the returned ball behind your far hip, allowing your body to recoil, and repeat the throw. Change direction and repeat reps on the other side. Start slowly and gradually increase the speed throughout the repetitions. Progress by increasing the distance between the catch and release point of the ball and lifting your heels slightly off the ground for the duration of the exercise.

Keep your core strong and your chest up throughout the movement.

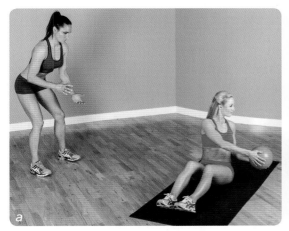 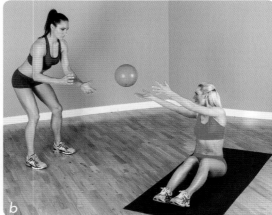

Figure 8.12 Seated side twist and throw.

REVERSE OVERHEAD THROW

Exercise Focus

Total-body explosive power

Equipment

2- to 5-kg medicine ball

How To

Check that the trajectory of your ball follows an arch. If the ball hits the floor too soon (i.e., before making contact with the wall), it is likely you are pulling it down at the release point rather than releasing it at the optimal point of extension.

Stand in an open space with 10 to 20 metres of space behind you, depending on your throwing ability. (If you have limited space or distance behind you, then work with a heavier ball, which is unlikely to travel as far.) With your feet wider than shoulder width, hold the medicine ball overhead with both hands (see figure 8.13*a*). Swing the ball down between your legs, bending your knees and keeping your back flat (see figure 8.13*b*). Extend from your knees and arms to throw the ball up and backwards over your head and then release it (see figure 8.13*c*), aiming for maximal distance. It is natural for you to travel backwards as you release the ball just be prepared to back step to catch yourself from stumbling over. Collect your ball and repeat.

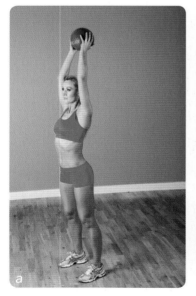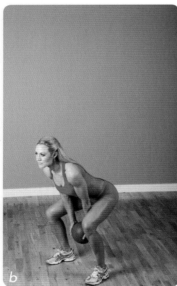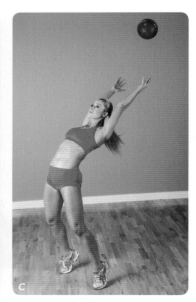

Figure 8.13   Reverse overhead throw.

SEATED VERTICAL THROW

Exercise Focus

Deltoid explosive power

Equipment

2- to 5-kg medicine ball

How To

Keep your core strong and your chest up to isolate your shoulders during the exercise.

Sit on the floor with your legs outstretched and hold the medicine ball at chest height. Turn your elbows out and position the ball with your palms facing upwards (see figure 8.14a). Extend at your elbows and fingertips to throw the ball directly overhead (see figure 8.14b). Catch it and repeat the movement. Progress by increasing the weight of the ball.

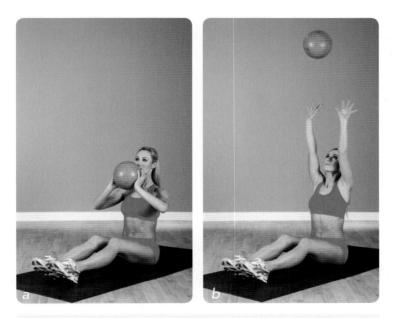

Figure 8.14   Seated vertical throw.

Olympic Lift Exercises

These exercises are the most comprehensive for total-body muscle activation and for developing maximum explosive power. They are not confined to the programme of a weightlifter, being utilised by athletes across numerous sports and disciplines, from marathon runners to track and field athletes and team sports players. One Olympic lift can do the work of several machines, achieving workout efficiency and saving time. If you want to make the most of your time in the gym, then learning these moves could be your time-saving solution to fitness.

To learn the correct technique prior to adding additional weight, begin by breaking the exercises down into their component parts, as we mentioned earlier in the chapter. Next, perform the sequence at about 50 to 60 percent maximal effort to allow your muscles, joints and neurological system to adapt and develop the correct motor learning process over the first couple of sessions. Repetitions and sets will vary depending on whether you are working for pure power or power endurance and you should also adjust the weight accordingly.

POWER CLEAN

Exercise Focus

Total-body power

Equipment

Lifting platform (or dedicated flat surface suitable for lifting), lifting bar (Olympic bar preferable), weight discs (vary weight according to strength and goal), and weights gloves (optional)

How To

Stand with your feet hip-width apart or slightly wider with the balls of your feet positioned under the bar. Squat down and hold the bar with an overhand grip slightly wider than shoulder width. Keep your back flat, chest up and hold your arms straight (see figure 8.15a).

To execute the movement, pull the bar up off the floor by extending your hips and knees. As the bar reaches your knees, vigorously raise your shoulders while keeping the barbell close to your thighs. As the bar passes the mid-thigh area, allow it to touch your thighs (see figure 8.15b). Continue to pull upwards, extending your body and moving onto your toes. Then, shrug your shoulders and pull the barbell upward with your arms, flexing your elbows out to the sides (see figure 8.15c). Quickly pull your body under the bar whilst rotating your elbows around the bar. Catch it on your shoulders as your knees bend to 90 degrees (see figure 8.15d). Stand up immediately to complete the repetition (see figure 8.15e). To lower the bar, bend your knees and drop it onto your thighs, and then lower it to the ground whilst keeping your back straight. If the weight is heavy, you may choose to drop the bar as you lower it.

Perform the movement smoothly and continuously, lifting steadily from the floor and then accelerating to the highest point of the movement. Avoid jerking the bar from the floor, as this will disrupt the movement pattern and potentially risk injury.

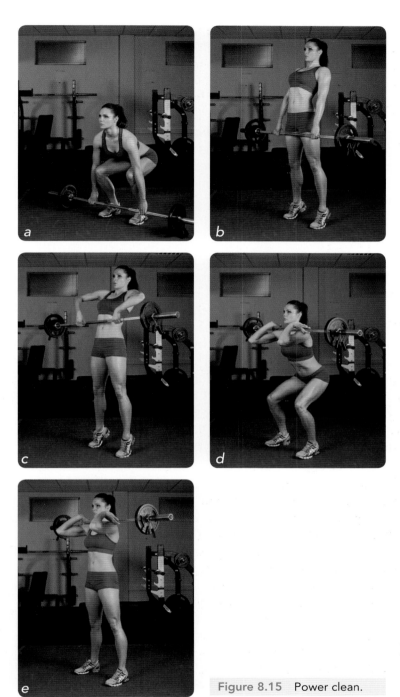

Figure 8.15   Power clean.

CLEAN AND JERK

Exercise Focus

Total-body power

Equipment

Lifting platform (or dedicated flat surface suitable for lifting), lifting bar (Olympic bar preferable), weight discs (vary weight according to strength and goal), and weights gloves (optional)

> *Most women can clean more weight than they can jerk, so you may require a lighter weight to that with which you performed the isolated power clean. Furthermore, shoulder stability is key to a successful jerk, so condition your shoulders with strength work prior to trying out this exercise.*

How To

Perform the clean movement as described previously (see figure 8.15a-e). Execute the jerk from the finish position of the clean. With the pressure on your heels, dip your body by bending your knees and ankles slightly (see figure 8.16a). Explosively drive upwards with your legs, pressing and splitting one foot forwards and the other backwards as quickly as possible while vigorously extending your arms overhead (see figure 8.16b). In the split position, your front shin should be vertical to the floor and your front foot flat with your back knee bent. The position of the bar should be directly over your ears, held at arm's length with your back straight. Push up with both legs and position your feet side by side to complete the movement (see figure 8.16c). To return the bar, lower it to your shoulders, bend your knees and then lower the bar to the ground or drop it, as per the return movement of the previous power clean exercise.

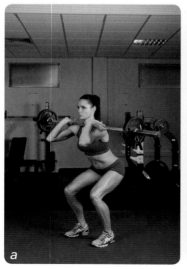
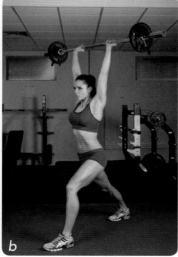
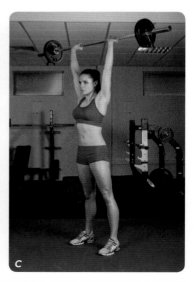

Figure 8.16   Clean and jerk.

SNATCH

Exercise Focus

Total-body power

Equipment

Lifting platform (or dedicated flat surface suitable for lifting), lifting bar (Olympic bar preferable), weight discs (varyweight according to strength and goal), and weights gloves (optional)

How To

Stand with your feet hip-width apart or slightly wider with the balls of your feet positioned under the bar. Squat down and hold the bar with a wide overhand grip. Arch your back, keep your chest up and arms straight (see figure 8.17a).

To execute the movement, pull the bar up off the floor by extending your hips and knees. As the bar reaches your knees, keep your back arched, maintaining the same angle to the floor as for your starting position. When the barbell passes your knees, vigorously raise your shoulders whilst keeping the bar as close to your legs as possible and as the bar passes your upper thighs, allow it to touch them. Continue to pull the bar upwards, extending your body (see figure 8.17b).

Next, shrug your shoulders and pull the barbell upwards with your arms, elbows out, and over the bar for as long as possible (see figure 8.17c). As the bar reaches its highest point, aggressively pull your body underneath the bar by dropping into a squat position and catching it at arm's length (see figure 8.17d). As soon as you have caught the barbell with locked-out arms in a squat position, stand up, keeping the barbell overhead, to complete the movement (see figure 8.17e). To return the bar, bend your knees slightly and lower the bar to rest on your mid-thighs. Then, move it to the ground, keeping a straight back. If the weight is heavy, and it is safe to do so, you can drop the bar from the finish position. This can reduce the stress and fatigue involved in lowering the bar when performing multiple sets.

Complete the snatch exercise as one complete continuous movement, lifting from the floor steadily and then accelerating to the top position.

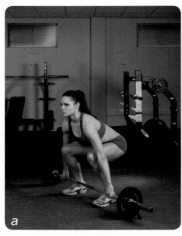
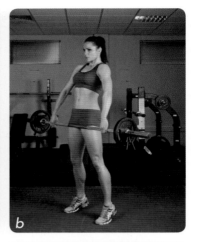
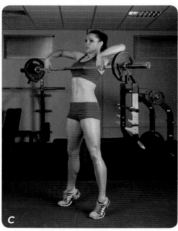
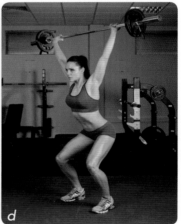
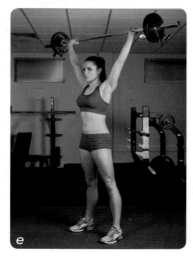

Figure 8.17   Snatch.

VIBRATION TRAINING EXERCISES

Performing standard strength exercises on a vibration plate, such as a Power Plate machine can simultaneously improve your power. This is because of the Tonic Vibration Reflex (TVR) created by holding a pre-tensed position (such as a squat position) combined with vibration. This TVR results in a much higher percentage of muscle fibre recruitment and better muscular coordination compared to ground based exercises without vibration. Furthermore, with vibration, your muscles are stimulated to contract at an accelerated speed as a result of a reflex response in your muscles. So although you are not jumping or bounding on the machine, as you would for conventional power training, your muscles still experience the stretch-shortening cycle, and power adaptations take place. This makes vibration training a great choice if you want to improve power but reduce the impact on your joints, such as when recovering from injury or when your goal is to maintain explosive power during a competitive sports season without the risk of injury. Hundreds of conventional strength exercises can be performed on a vibration platform and these include squats, lunges, press-ups and triceps dips, to mention just a few. You can perform these exercises either statically or dynamically.

Sled Sprint Exercises

Sprinting is a classic example of power in action. You can perform your sprints on an ergometer machine (treadmill, rower, stationary bike or elliptical), on the track, on grass, up hills and in the pool. The principle behind a sprint is to perform each movement pattern maximally and repeatedly for a short, set distance (short-term power). A strong core, good total-body strength and good technique will improve your sprinting performance and efficiency. For examples of power endurance sprint workouts, please see chapter 6: Go Anaerobic. Sprinting typically involves your body weight alone, but you can execute sprints with additional loads to further enhance your power and force output. Remember, force equals mass times acceleration! You can perform sled sprints by either pulling a sled (or person) so the load is behind you or pushing a sled (or car or person) so the load is in front of you.

SLED PULL SPRINT

Exercise Focus

Total-body speed and power

Equipment

Small sled and a harness (or simply loop a rope or harness directly through a weighted disc with a hole where the weight bar typically inserts or around the waist of a partner) and a flat, smooth surface.

How To

Place your arms in the shoulder harness or simply tie the attached ropes around your waist and face away from the weighted sled, or your partner, in a standing or three-point sprint start position. Assume a forward lean position, and then quickly accelerate, striking the ground with your toes in short, fast movements as you build up speed and knee drive. If using a partner they will need to lean backwards and apply a breaking force in the opposite direction in which you are pulling them. To progress, you can increase the sled weight, your partner's resistance or your sprint distance.

Your body should remain in a slight forward lean position for the duration of the 30-metre sprint to avoid the weight of the sled pulling you backwards. Keep your ankles, knees and hips strong and pump your arms to generate more power and momentum.

SLED OR CAR PUSH SPRINT

Exercise Focus

Lower body speed and power

Equipment

A metal frame sled device, small car (with handbrake off) or partner. Preferably, you will have a partner to steer the car or to act as a moving sled, pushing back to apply resistance as you push him or her along.

How To

Stand facing the sled, car, or partner. Hold the sled handles, place your hands against the car or place your hands on the back of your partner. Keep your arms straight. To initiate the movement, rapidly lean your body weight into the sled/car/person by dropping your body downwards and raising your heels off the ground. Drive your knees forwards, contacting the ground with short rapid steps whilst keeping your weight low behind your sled. To progress, increase the weight of your sled device or, if using a partner, ask him or her to apply more resistance back against you.

Although you are eaning forwards, do not allow your hips to drift too far backwards, or you will reduce the force being transferred through your body to your sled.

ADDITIONAL POWER TRAINING EXERCISE SUGGESTIONS

In addition to the preceding power training exercises, you might also want to explore and try the following modes for power training.

Cable Machine Exercises

The cable machine is a great way to incorporate power exercises into your gym-based workout. The exercises are performed in a small space and the movement direction is determined by the machine, so it is a safe and controlled environment. Cable power exercises include wood chops, turn and punch, knee drives (using the ankle straps) and side turn rotations. For each exercise, accelerate the cable from start to finish position.

Kettlebell Exercises

The shape of a kettlebell and its custom-made handle makes it ideal for acceleration movements through a swinging action. You can add a power dimension to any circuit training workout by incorporating the following kettlebell exercises: dead-lift swings, single-arm snatch and pelvic bridge pull-overs.

Boxing Exercises

These exercises are fast and powerful and thus fantastic for all-round conditioning and achieving a high calorie burn. They also specifically help develop strength and power in the upper body, which is often lacking in women. Exercises include the basic jab, cross and hook. Perform these for a set period of time or number of repetitions and experiment with exercise combinations.

AT A GLANCE

- Power is defined as strength expressed at high speed. It is the body's preferred method for generating force. Both sport and everyday activities rely on the generation of power for optimal performance and efficiency, so training for power has numerous benefits.

- Power movements rely on the recruitment of a large number of muscle fibres and the predominant use of your fast-twitch muscle fibres.

- The many benefits to increasing your power include increased fitness in a short workout time; increased muscle tone and definition; increased metabolism and fat burning; increased release of testosterone, human growth hormone and serotonin for adaptation, repair and regeneration; fun and variety and improved sporting performance.

- The two main types of power include pure explosive power (the ability to produce a single maximal explosive action) and power endurance (the ability to produce repeated power movements with minimal loss of force).

- Prior to attempting power training, condition your body for the impact and intensity that is required with general strength conditioning and joint stability work. Also, break down any complex power moves into their component parts before performing them at full speed and intensity.

- Recommended power-training workouts include body-weight plyometrics, bounding, box jump plyometrics, medicine ball power exercises, Olympic lifts and sled sprints.

- The average fitness enthusiast can include a power endurance workout one or two times every 7 to 10 days and a pure power workout once per week. A competitive athlete should phase in and adapt power training according to her current training phase and competition schedule.

9

Get Agile

In its simplest form, agility describes the ability to change direction of body movement, incorporating elements of both acceleration and deceleration. At the highest levels of sporting performance, agility is a manifestation of the strength of the mind–body relationship, resulting in the body moving in total harmony with and at the limits of its own structural design. Mostly, agility training is focused on speed work rather than conditioning. It teaches motor skills with the aim of developing the ability to accommodate intense neural work, even when approaching fatigue. In competition situations, elite sportswomen may need to execute precise movement patterns in just a couple of seconds. It's not just exclusively for the sports domain, however. Agility training will place new demands on your body, helping you not only increase your fitness, but also develop skills that you can transfer to work, rest and play. If in your downtime you partake in activities such as martial arts, tennis, netball, lacrosse and football, you can expect to see your game improve.

Since agility training usually relies on short bouts of high-intensity effort, it can be a truly effective route to both losing weight and improving general fitness. Training can be very varied and, therefore, a lot more fun than simply running in straight lines or repetitively lifting something up and down in the gym. An additional by-product is decreased risk of injury as you condition your body for changes in direction and stimuli. So, it's got to be worth adding to your routine.

COMPONENTS OF AGILITY

Agility is a crucial performance component in most sports and is an expression of the combined forces of speed, power and skill. It encompasses many demands, from the tennis player's lateral movement to the high jumper's ability to transfer horizontal to vertical force as he or she approaches the bar for takeoff, and from the tae kwon do player's hand–foot co-ordination to the fencer's escape and riposte tactics. Regardless of the sport, practice will improve this often underrated commodity.

Before getting into the mechanics of the workouts, let's take a look at what we actually mean when we talk about agility by breaking it down to its constituent parts:

- *Balance*—The ability to maintain static and dynamic equilibrium of both the limbs and the body as a whole.
- *Co-ordination*—The ability to perform a range of simple to complex movements with precision timing, sequence and continuity.
- *Reaction*—The ability to recruit neuromuscular responses with minimal time delay in response to visual, auditory or kinaesthetic stimulus.
- *Spatial awareness*—The degree of control one has over the body in space.
- *Rhythm*—The skill of matching movement to time.
- *Kinaesthetic sense*—The awareness of tension in the muscles during movement that helps to adjust and improve execution.
- *Movement selection*—The ability to choose appropriate movement patterns to accommodate actual and perceived demands.

Multidirectional exercises require these components to work in harmony, rather than in isolation, as they are closely linked. In addition, although earlier we declared agility training to be speed work rather than conditioning, a basic platform of strength (particularly in your legs) is a prerequisite for performing the drills effectively. This is why elite sportswomen dedicate a period of their preseason training purely to conditioning workouts.

Improving your agility is an incremental process beginning with the development of locomotion skills, which starts during children's play when they try to avoid being caught by their friends in school playground games. Initially, movement is inefficient, as arm motion is awkward, balance is questionable and co-ordination is lacking. Learning basic motor skills is the first stage, therefore, with variation in drills being the best way to learn a good foundation of general movement patterns. If you've never attempted agility training before, you may wish to begin with the following:

- Perform stationary arm movements, such as pumping the arms while the feet are fixed.
- Practise the running motion with one leg while keeping the other in contact with the floor.
- Jumping in place to a set rhythm is also a great way to get started, so try this with different tunes playing on your MP3 to vary the tempo.
- Perform balance exercises such as simply standing on one leg or hopping.

- Practise direction change, starting with curved patterns such as running around cones in the studio or trees in the park in a figure-of-eight pattern. Next, move on to sharp changes in direction that require a stop-and-start pattern. The key concept to grasp here is to decelerate by using multiple short steps rather than a long braking stride to reduce shearing forces in your knees.

- There exist a number of protocols to measure agility, including the Illinois, T-drill, hexagonal and stork-stand tests. One of the most common is the simple ladder run, in which you time the speed you need to cover the 20-rung obstacle (one foot in each gap). A time of less than 3.4 seconds is rated as excellent. A good idea is to test yourself every 12 weeks to monitor your progress.

AGILITY TRAINING METHODS

Since the primary application for agility training is in preparation for many sports, trainers usually analyse the basic game-time demands of specific sports and then create challenges that mirror such. The aims of agility training are to enhance body control, increase the ability to overcome inertia, improve footwork and master directional change. These factors can be improved simultaneously through multidirectional drills involving stops and starts, often performed at speed. An important maxim to observe dictates that you should be comfortable with the exercises before working to fatigue, so incorporate agility exercises into your warm-ups and cooldowns for a short while in order to become familiar with them before attempting an intense agility-training workout. Try some of the great drills described in chapter 4 that specifically address movements for warming-up and cooling-down.

LINEAR PACE CHANGE

Exercise Focus

Reaction

How To

Begin with a jog, and then alternate the speed to run and then to sprint. Shift up through your gears smoothly and then go back down again.

Add a random element by reacting to a particular word in a song you're listening to. For example, speed up to a run for 30 seconds if you hear the word 'move' or sprint for 10 seconds if you hear the word 'fast'. Ideally, choose a few common words so you can guarantee they will come up fairly regularly.

HULA HOOPING

Exercise Focus

Co-ordination and rhythm

Equipment

Hula hoop

How To

Stand inside the hoop with one foot in front of the other. Lift the hoop to just above waist level, holding it against your back. Push the hoop around your waist and shift your weight forwards and backwards. Work in both directions, although you may find you have a stronger side so ensure your weaker side is tested too.

Try to avoid circling your hips. Think more of rocking or pumping.

POWER HOPPING

Exercise Focus

Balance and kinaesthetic sense

How To

Start at a specific spot and then hop forwards, backwards, side to side and on diagonals. Always keep your body facing in the same direction. Try to focus on bouncing as opposed to jerking movements, landing on the ball of your foot and bending your knee. Learning to decelerate and accelerate leads to more efficient movement patterns and control of force production.

The bend of the knee before the next hop is known as a countermove (i.e., doing the opposite movement to prepare for an exertion exercise), which helps increase the natural elasticity of the muscle fascia.

ADDING AGILITY TRAINING TO YOUR WORKOUT

You can easily tweak the strength training exercises that you learned in chapter 7 to improve your kinaesthetic sense and spatial awareness:

- Perform standing exercises on just one leg for balance.
- Sit on a BOSU ball during upper body exercises to improve balance and kinaesthetic sense.
- Put one foot on a core board for squats or lunges to improve co-ordination and balance.
- Swap the chest press for press-ups with one or both hands on a medicine ball for balance.
- Use free weights rather than fixed machines and dumbbells rather than barbells to place a greater neuromuscular demand on your body for improving spatial awareness.
- Include lots of rotation exercises (e.g., Russian twist).
- Think laterally: Squats and lunges should be performed to the side and at diagonals rather than static, to the front and to the rear.

LADDER DRILL

Exercise Focus
Spatial awareness

Equipment
Soft ladder

How To
The primary aim of ladder drills is to improve speed, so work at high intensity. Consequently, you should allow a short rest between repetitions to allow yourself to perform the next one at full effort once again. You can employ ladder drills as a component within a training session or as a stand-alone workout. In the latter case, for a good 30-minute session, begin with a warm-up followed by 5 minutes on each of the preceding drills and then do a cool down.

As mentioned in the testing procedures, a floor ladder is a very useful tool, but don't feel that you have to invest in an expensive prop. You can easily make one at home if you have a bit of space and a roll of parcel tape. Lay down two parallel lines about 30 centimetres apart and then add the 20 rungs, spacing them 35 centimetres apart. Ladder exercises include the following:

High Knee Lift

Drive your elbows backwards to help increase speed and concentrate on getting your feet back on the ground as quickly as possible, picturing your legs as pistons. Land on the balls of your feet and keep your head and chest lifted.

Low Knee Lift

After running through the ladder, continue for 10 metres at full sprint, gradually lengthening your stride. Observe the same technique tips as in the previous exercise.

Lateral Step

Keep your hips low, stay on the balls of your feet, don't lift the feet up, and focus on sideways movement. Remember to work in both directions.

Lateral Shuffle

Face the length of the ladder and then shuffle across it by shifting your position: Begin with both feet on one side of the ladder, move both feet inside it, and then move again to place both feet on the other side. Make your way back to the starting side, but move one rung up the ladder. Continue shuffling from side to side and working your way up the ladder.

In–Out Jump

With your feet together, travel the length of the ladder, jumping into the space between the rungs then out to the sides again.

In–Out Hop

Travel the length of the ladder, jumping on one foot into the space between the rungs then out to the same side, remembering to work both left and right legs. On your left leg you will work up the left side of the ladder and vice-versa on the right leg. Focus on landing softly by bending your knee as you touch down, using the thigh muscles to absorb the impact.

Ski Jumps

Start at the side of the ladder with your feet together and facing the ladder at a 45-degree angle, your knees bent and your arms drawn back. Now explode upwards, swinging your arms to help gain momentum, and jump across the ladder. Turn your lower body as you cross to the other side and land with your feet again facing slightly towards the ladder.

CUTTING

Exercise Focus

Reaction

How To

You can perform these drills in any open space, using markers such as cones, plastic cups, stones or even trees and lampposts. Perform them at sprint speed, quickly recovering between each repetition for 10 to 15 seconds. Do 10 repetitions of each drill to get familiar with the movement and then execute it with precision, efficiency and control as you begin to fatigue. Cutting exercises include the following:

Linear Runs

Run forwards to touch the marker and then backwards to your start point. These are sprints, so keep the distance to around 10 metres.

Lateral Runs

Cover the distance between two markers placed 20 metres apart by running sideways, alternately crossing the rear foot over the front one and then behind it again.

Slalom

Run along a line of markers set 5 metres apart, weaving between them with smooth movements. Try not to lose speed as you encounter each obstacle.

Zigzag

Place markers in two lines 5 metres apart and staggered at 5-metre intervals in a zigzag pattern. Run from one to the next, changing direction as swiftly as possible. Remember to shorten your stride length in order to decelerate and then accelerate away from the pivot point.

Square

Place markers in roughly a 10-metre square formation, and then run around them. Face the same way throughout the circuit so that you run forwards, to the side, backwards and then to the other side.

SKIPPING

Exercise Focus

Co-ordination and rhythm

Equipment

Buy a quality rope (rather than a kids' version) that will last through repeated workouts and help you achieve an even swing. The rope should be long enough to reach your armpits when you stand in the middle of the loop.

How To

Make sure you have enough space that you won't hit anything (or anyone) with the rope. Land softly after each jump. Make contact with the ball of your foot first, and then roll through the lateral arch to your heels. This is the reverse of the foot action used in jogging. Skipping exercises include the following:

Basic Skip

Hold a handle in each hand and let the rope rest on the floor behind your heels. Keep the hands at hip level and use the wrists, not the shoulders, to swing the rope overhead and down to the feet. As the rope approaches, keep your feet together and jump only a few centimetres off the ground as it passes underneath you. Land on the balls of your feet as softly as possible. Repeat this process slowly at first, and then try to find a steady rhythm. If you struggle to time your jump, make the rope hit the ground a foot or so in front of you before jumping. The noise of the rope hitting the floor will help you time your jump.

Crossover

Start with the basic skip. When the rope is directly above your head, cross your arms at your waist. As the rope approaches the floor, hop over it. Once it's overhead again, uncross your arms so that they're back in the starting position. Keep your wrists firm at all times and your hands low and pulled in close. The crossover works best if you cross and uncross the arms every other jump (i.e., alternating crossed jumps with the basic skip).

Side to Side

Hop from side to side as the rope passes under your feet, covering about 15 centimetres to each side. Keep the knees and ankles soft to avoid injury.

Twist

As you jump up, twist at the waist, moving your legs and feet 45 degrees to the side while keeping the torso facing forward. Concentrate on keeping your feet together throughout the movement. On the next swing, jump and twist again, this time moving your legs and feet to a similar position on the other side. To make this easier, you may wish to slow the pace and jump a little higher. To avoid knee injuries, ensure that the whole length of your leg (and not just the lower leg) turns with you.

Jog

Rest the rope on the floor behind your heels and lift your right foot a few centimetres off the floor, resting your weight on the left foot. Begin as in the basic skip, but hop on the left foot. Hop 8 times on the left, and then change to the right foot. Once you're comfortable, lower the number to 4 hops, then 2 and finally 1.

Skipping Jacks

Begin with your basic skip and then jump a little higher, landing with your feet about hip-width apart. On the next jump, return your feet to the centre. Avoid landing with your feet too far apart, as they could get tangled in the rope.

REACTION BALL

Exercise Focus

Reaction and movement selection

Equipment

Reaction ball (irregularly shaped ball that has a knobbly surface to produce a random bounce, even when thrown at flat surfaces)

How To

Stand a few metres from a wall, throw the ball at it and then try to catch it as it bounces back. Don't worry if you miss it; retrieving it and returning to your start mark as quickly as possible is all part of the exercise. For additional challenge, throw the ball at an uneven surface, such as a tree trunk.

You can make your own reaction ball quite easily and cheaply. Purchase a children's bouncy ball, the solid rubber type. Using the sharp end of a potato peeler, carefully dig out a couple of chunks so that the surface is no longer spherical. The ball should now bounce at unpredictable angles. For the simplest approach, however, you could use a rugby ball, which will also produce random bounces that force you to react.

Improving your speed of reaction enables you to respond first to an opportunity to attack before it disappears and also to recognise the opponent's manoeuvre so you can defend before it's too late. When training, then, always work at maximum speed.

AT A GLANCE

- Agility is the ability to change the direction of body movement while incorporating elements of both acceleration and deceleration.
- It incorporates balance, co-ordination, reaction, spatial awareness, rhythm, kinaesthetic sense and movement selection.
- It is a vital component of skill-related fitness for most sportswomen.
- For the recreational exerciser, agility training can relieve the boredom of regular workouts and reduce the risk of injury.
- A basic level of strength is required. Since most of the drills focus on speed, they are usually performed at a high intensity.

10

Personalise Your Programme

At times, individual circumstances and demands make life, particularly working out, more of a challenge. This chapter aims to investigate a few of those challenges and to pre-warn (and therefore pre-arm) you to accommodate them. A number of genuine issues apply specifically to women, but forethought and planning will ensure these do not throw your workout programme off track. We firmly believe that fitness is for life. Here is some vital advice for overcoming some of the challenges you might face on your fitness journey.

TRAINING DURING MENSTRUATION

Water retention is common during menstruation, and it can leave you feeling bloated. Your energy levels may be low, and a general feeling of discomfort can push exercise down your list of priorities. However, sometimes just getting to the start line can be enough. If you give it a try, you will find that the instant buzz and endorphin release from exercise energises you. You will be able to complete your workout, feeling all the better for doing so. Furthermore, the increase in blood flow during exercise leads to an increase in lymph flow, which in turn reduces water retention. It's wise to moderate your workout intensity a little bit if you're feeling particularly lethargic. Be sure to drink plenty of fluids. If you really are on a low, turn this into a gentle exercise day by opting for a swim. The water will reduce stress on your lower back, which might be suffering. Alternatively, try a yoga class, as some poses have been reported to help relieve cramps. The breathing exercises can also reduce tension, particularly in the neck and shoulders, as well as help to calm the nervous system.

Refuelling at this time requires special attention, as blood loss can contribute to low iron levels. This causes the feelings of lethargy, since iron transports oxygen around your body to power the muscle cells. Good sources of this vital nutrient are spinach, beans, raisins, tofu, apricots and fortified cereals. Fish contains linoleic acid, which can help ease cramping, and fresh fruit and vegetables can also be of benefit as they are low in sodium, so helping to reduce water retention.

Research shows that using an oral contraceptive can help to maintain hormone levels and so counter the fluctuations at this time that reduce the ability to train effectively. Certainly this is worth consideration for the serious competitor, as is the obvious step of scheduling races around your menstrual cycle if this is an option.

AVOIDING THE FEMALE ATHLETE TRIAD

The *female athlete triad* describes the combination of three related aspects that lead to an unhealthy situation, namely disordered eating, amenorrhea and osteoporosis.

Disordered eating refers to the many, often unhealthy, eating routines that people, particularly women, follow in an attempt to control weight. They may have unrealistic goals that often result from perceived pressure from friends, family, society or sports coaches. Sportswomen in certain disciplines are more at risk, with dancing, swimming, gymnastics and running placing a specific emphasis on lean aesthetics. Additional common contributory factors include family issues, poor knowledge of nutrition and low self-esteem. A combination of some, or even all, of these factors can lead to extreme calorie restriction, forced vomiting and use of medication such as laxatives and diuretics. Sadly, disordered eating not only impairs your ability to work out, thus slowing your progress towards your goals, but also hurts your health status by affecting the cardiovascular, endocrine and thermoregulatory systems.

From a very basic viewpoint, insufficient calorie intake obviously leads to reduced energy stores in the body, particularly muscle glycogen. So, your ability to exercise at high intensities, a concept we've repeatedly recommended throughout this book, will be severely limited. You will also be less likely to achieve the very results you train for. Sadly, lack of sufficient calorie intake can be the precursor to the second component of the female athlete triad, amenorrhea (cessation of menstruation). This is thought to happen in two ways. First, exercise stress can potentially keep the hypothalamus from secreting the gonadotrophin-releasing hormone that stimulates the beginning of the menstrual cycle. Second, with so few fuel stores available, the body sacrifices reproduction in order to use the energy so the vital organs can continue to perform. Fortunately, simply increasing food intake will lead to a return to normal menstruation.

The final of the three components is osteoporosis, which is caused by reduced oestrogen levels associated with amenorrhea. The condition warrants greater investigation due to its prevalence within the female population worldwide. Bone growth begins in the foetus as calcium and magnesium salts are deposited and built up, a process known as ossification. Remodelling continues through life as osteoblast cells deposit mineral salts to promote new bone growth and old bone tissue gets broken down and absorbed by osteoclast cells, releasing calcium, potassium and phosphate compounds into the blood stream. In childhood, bone formation outpaces reabsorption, resulting in increased length and width of the bones, but the reverse is true in later years. Peak bone mass is achieved at around 25 years of age.

The flow of calcium in and out of the bone tissue is controlled by calcitriol, which is formed in the kidneys in a process where vitamin D (absorbed from sunlight) is a key ingredient. The parathyroid gland controls the kidney secretions so that if calcium levels in the blood fall below a certain point, more will automatically be released. This balancing act is assisted by the presence of oestrogen. The drop in oestrogen levels associated with the female athlete triad results in greater bone reabsorption and so the loss of bone density. As no obvious outward signs of bone health exist, you may not know your bones have lost density until you suffer a fracture following a relatively minor trauma. The most common fracture sites are the wrist, hip and vertebrae.

The risk of osteoporosis is increased by a number of factors:

- *Family history*—Daughters of mothers who have suffered the disease are likely to possess a lower bone density.
- *Ethnic background*—Afro-Caribbean and Hispanic people show less likelihood of suffering than European and Asian individuals.
- *Age*—Bone mineral density generally declines with increasing years due to the reduction in osteoblast activity.
- *Medical history*—Sufferers of rheumatoid arthritis, hyperthyroidism, Crohn's disease and coeliac disease all have an increased chance of osteoporosis.
- *Alcohol use*—The diuretic effect of drinking removes vital supplies of calcium in the urine, which slows the growth of new bone.
- *Smoking habits*—Smoking decreases oestrogen levels in the blood stream, leading to a reduction in the amount of calcium absorbed by the bones.

You can deploy two key strategies to reduce your chance of becoming another osteoporosis statistic. The first is to manage your diet. Foods containing calcium positively influence bone mineral density. As established earlier, low calcium intake will lead the body to reabsorb bone tissue in order to maintain adequate blood calcium levels. Low-fat dairy and leafy green vegetables provide a direct route to obtaining the calcium we need. In addition, consuming fruit and vegetables, specifically those that are more alkaline, reduces the amount of calcium lost in urine and therefore also has a positive influence on bone density. The second strategy is getting plenty of exercise. Since bone adapts to the mechanical stresses applied to it, then loading of the bones through physical activity will lead to positive changes in structure. Exercise has been shown to improve bone density at any age.

Of these two tactics, exercise carries the greatest potential to affect bone mass, as it both produces gravitational force on the skeleton and loads muscles, effects which have been proven to promote bone health. More specifically, resistance training is a vital component that must be part of your training routine. The reason strength training works is because the skeleton responds adaptively to forces applied to it. If stress is beyond a certain threshold, cell activity changes to stimulate an increase in strength of the bone. This occurs through a phenomenon known as the *piezoelectric principle,* a term that comes from the Greek translation of the word 'squeeze', which helps us understand how it links to the performance of strength exercises. The tendon of a muscle exerts mechanical stress on its point of attachment to the bone, causing a charge to be released from within the collagen fibres. This voltage then attracts the oppositely charged osteoblasts that we talked about earlier, which deposit minerals at the site. The result, then, is a localised increase in bone density.

It is most important to understand that cardio training is not as effective as strength training for preventing osteoporosis. So, if your programme is geared toward improving your running, swimming or cycling performance, you really need to add regular resistance sessions. Also, the bone-loading effect is site specific, so it's vital to follow a whole-body approach to strength training.

WORKING OUT WHEN PREGNANT

Exercise is important both before and after giving birth for helping to reduce pregnancy symptoms, control weight gain and ease labour. It also tones the stretched pelvic floor and abdominal muscles, plus realigns posture. Paula Radcliffe, who won the New York Marathon only 10 months after her first child was born, is rumoured to have run 14 miles (23 km) each day when expecting her second child. The truth is that training is very much down to the individual and even to the specific pregnancy, as symptoms can vary for a woman from one to the next.

Workout Modifications During Pregnancy

As many of you know, pregnancy is made up of three phases of roughly equal duration, characterized by the changes that occur in the body at these times. Your training will need to be adapted for these periods, so let's take a moment to consider such.

General guidelines for exercise during pregnancy are as follows:

- Aim for two or three workouts per week.
- If you are not a regular exerciser already, work at low intensity.
- Drink plenty of water.
- Keep your movements smooth, never ballistic or bouncing.
- After 20 weeks, avoid exercises where you lie flat on your back. This is due to the risk of supine hypotensive syndrome, where the weight of the baby rests on the main blood vessels, possibly restricting the blood flow to both you and the baby.
- Focus on constant, relaxed breathing.
- Limit your range of motion.

Fatigue and nausea are common symptoms in the first trimester, but you will likely be able to comfortably continue your level of exercise. Listen to your body and rest if necessary, particularly as miscarriage is most common towards the end of this phase. However, exercise is not thought to be a cause.

In the second trimester, the blood volume, body weight and levels of the hormone relaxin increase. The first signs of the tummy expanding can also be seen. Morning sickness usually subsides, although occasionally it continues through the full term.

The third trimester can bring symptoms of breathlessness plus posture and balance issues, depending on the amount of weight gained and where the baby is being carried in the abdomen. The higher levels of relaxin can also destabilise the joints.

This information enables us to appreciate how workouts during pregnancy should be modified.

Warm-Ups During Pregnancy

The extra load on the cardiovascular system caused by the increased blood volume will increase your heart rate, so always begin gently. This will also reduce risks associated with joint stability issues. The shift of your centre of gravity may make changes in speed of movement and direction more difficult, so build up gradually. Since your body temperature will already be elevated, this section of your session can be shorter than normal.

Cardio Training During Pregnancy

As pregnancy can reduce proprioception and therefore agility, avoid agility exercises, particularly later in the pregnancy. Whilst you can maintain your cardio training in the first trimester, reduce the impact starting in the second trimester in light of changes in the pelvic floor and decreased joint stability. Since your heart rate will already be higher than usual, you will not need to work as hard to achieve a training effect. Your workload must remain below the anaerobic threshold as lactic acid builds up, as this can be an issue for the growing baby. Your working pulse shouldn't exceed 70 percent maximum (calculated by subtracting your age from 220), and a 20-minute session is the ideal duration. Energy levels can be a problem, so regularly consume small portions of complex carbohydrate.

Strength Training During Pregnancy

Concentrate on perfect technique during resistance exercises, as instability within the joints may put you at greater risk of injury due to poor alignment or movement patterns. Additionally, avoid static isometric exercises such as the plank, as these may lead to an increase in blood pressure. Exercises where you lie flat on your back are not recommended from around 20 weeks, as mentioned earlier. Once the baby starts to show with an extended tummy, avoid traditional abdominal exercises, which put stress on muscles that are already being stretched and weakened. They may also exacerbate the diastasis, or separation, of the fibrous tissue that runs down the middle of the abdomen.

Flexibility Training During Pregnancy

The increased level of the hormone relaxin means you need to take care when performing stretching exercises. If you push the positions too far, your ligaments may slacken and remain loose after the birth, leading to unstable joints. Interestingly, this is more of an issue during repeated pregnancies. A number of stretching exercises will be more difficult due to the size and position of the developing baby and possibly due to increased body fat, so experiment with different positions to find comfortable options.

Pregnancy is actually a great time to think about expanding your exercise horizons and trying something different that you may not have considered previously but is better suited to you at the moment. As the weight of the growing baby increases, aqua workouts become more appealing. The water's buoyancy reduces stress in the pelvic floor and joints, particularly helping the lower back, and makes reduced-impact jogging possible. An extra bonus is that the resistance of the water against your moving limbs produces a toning effect for your muscles. Regarding dry-land options, brisk walking and yoga are good choices. The latter increases joint stability and provides breathing techniques that could possibly be useful during labour. Most yoga centres do specific pregnancy classes.

Exercising Safely During Pregnancy

Let's now consider some specific exercises with tips to ensure you work out safely and effectively at this important time:

- Control squats so that the heels always remain in firm contact with the floor to provide stability. Also, concentrate on evenly spreading the weight rather than favouring one leg, as this can stress the sacroiliac joint where the bottom of the spine links to the pelvis.
- To reduce the risk of lower back issues, support yourself during side bends, control trunk rotation and avoid hyperextension.
- Perform standing leg lifts with a focus on centring the pelvis, as shifting side to side can cause problems for the symphysis pubis joint at the bottom of the pelvis.
- Restrict abdominal exercises to pelvic tilts and hip hitches.
- Pelvic floor muscles are vital, so contract them by visualizing pulling front to back and vice-versa. Concentrate on relaxing the muscles in the abdomen and thighs. Try holding contractions for around 8 seconds to improve endurance and pulsing to improve control.
- Perform standing exercises and seated positions with the knees bent, as straight legs can cause the hamstrings to pull the pelvis into a tilt that stresses the lumbar spine.

SPECIFIC ANTE-NATAL EXERCISE CONSIDERATIONS

Various factors might affect your motivation to maintain an exercise routine during pregnancy, so remember that the benefits of working out can be more than purely physical:

- *Confidence*—Some women appear radiant during pregnancy, whilst others can struggle with the extra responsibility and fears of a negative effect on their lifestyle. The endorphin release from exercise will give you that feel-good boost just when you need it most.

- *Clothing*—Regular workout attire will not fit as well once weight begins to creep up, so purchase loose items so you feel comfortable when exercising.

- *Me time*—Morning sickness, other children and work can all get in the way of your workouts, so plan your me time regularly.

Postnatal Exercise

Once your baby is born, you will probably be raring to get back into exercise, but you can't simply go full steam ahead; you will need to build up to your previous level of fitness incrementally. Let's take a moment to explain why. Even if you did happen to have the energy to begin in the first months after birth, you probably shouldn't engage in exercise until after the standard 6-week examination, when the body has returned to its former status in terms of many of the biological changes that occurred during pregnancy. Relaxin levels have usually reduced considerably by this point, so working on stability by using free weights exercises, rather than machines, is a good idea. Be aware, however, that it will take months for the relaxin to totally leave your system, so it's even more important at this time to concentrate on correct technique.

After birth, your centre of gravity will shift back towards normal. Take time to refamiliarise yourself with your neutral spine position, as this should be fixed when doing resistance exercises to protect your lower spine. Weight loss will occur naturally, usually taking anywhere between 3 and 12 months, but cardio workouts will definitely speed this process. Low impact should still be the choice for cardio, so get in the pool or try brisk walking and low-intensity aerobics.

Your abdominal wall could stretch as much as 8 inches (20 cm) in length and an incredible 20 inches (50 cm) in width, so start engaging the area as soon as possible. If you experienced abdominal diastasis, you will need time for it to repair. This could take place within days, but it is more likely to take weeks, hence the 6-week threshold mentioned earlier. Start with isometric, or static, contractions whilst lying on your back and also whilst on all fours, such as Klapps crawls (see following section). Once you begin to notice the return of strength and definition to the abdominal muscles and reduced separation, you can move on to sit-ups and similar exercises. Following a caesarean birth, however, avoid exercise until after the 12-week check-up.

KLAPPS CRAWLS

Exercise Focus

Abdominal and lower back muscles

How To

Assume an all-fours position, with the hands shoulder-width apart and knees hip-width apart. Place the hands directly under the shoulders and the knees directly under the hips. Aim for 5 repetitions (to each side as necessary), focusing on smooth, controlled movement and working to your full range of comfortable motion on each of the following exercises:

1. Pull your navel in tightly, rounding your lower back. At the same time, look down at the floor (see figure 10.1a).

2. Next, actively press your tummy towards the floor and lift your head to look up to the ceiling (see figure 10.1b).

3. Keeping your hips fixed in position and resisting the temptation to sit back on your heels, walk your hands around to one side (see figure 10.1c) and then back to the starting position. Repeat to the other side.

4. Reach one hand as far under your body as you can (see figure 10.1d), then bring it back and continue the movement to lift your hand towards the ceiling (see figure 10.1e). Fix your gaze on the moving hand throughout the exercise.

5. Draw one knee towards the elbow of the opposite arm (see figure 10.1f), and then lift that arm and reach it forward, simultaneously lifting and stretching the moving leg out behind, in a Superman position (see figure 10.1g).

6. Return both your arm and leg to the ground, keep your upper body fixed and your abdominal muscles engaged, and shift your hips from side to side in a swinging motion (see figure 10.1h).

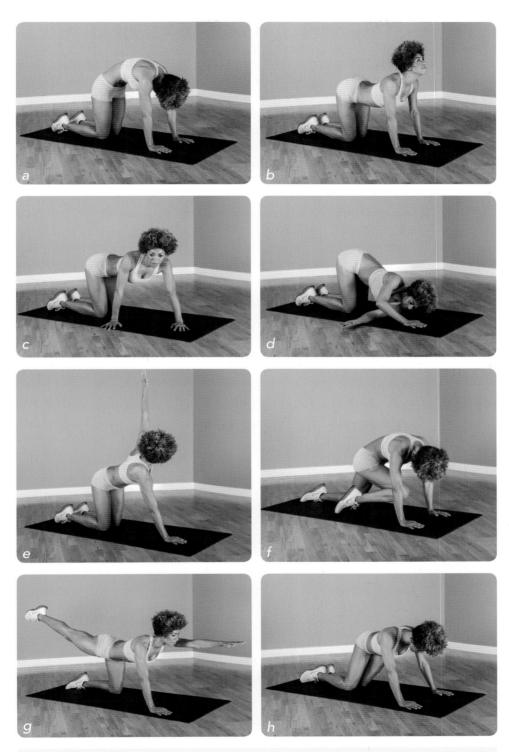

Figure 10.1 Klapps crawls.

STRENGTHENING TO REDUCE INJURIES

Having read this far, you are aware that your fitness level improves when adaptive physiological changes follow a training session, a principle known as *supercompensation*. As an example, your muscles absorb more protein, so enabling you to generate greater force. To keep moving towards your goals, you need to keep increasing the workload as your cardiorespiratory capacity improves and your muscles strengthen. However, you can risk a number of injuries if you constantly push your body to the limits, so equip yourself with tactics to help reduce the risk of being sidelined.

Unfortunately, a gender difference exists when it comes to training injuries, specifically to the knee, as a result of the variation in structure of the male and female skeletons. Women's hips are proportionally wider for childbirth purposes. As a result, the angle the thigh makes with the shin, known as the Q-angle, is greater for women than for men. This is suggested as the reason that relatively more females record injury to the anterior cruciate ligament, the band of connective tissue that crosses the knee joint, giving it stability. Another concern is the fact that women usually have a greater degree of anterior pelvis tilt than men. Therefore, women should strengthen the glutes and stretch the hip flexors to help to realign the pelvis, as well as strengthen the quadriceps to stabilise the knee joint. The following exercises are proposed for dealing with this issue:

- Rear lunge with upper body rotation (see figure 10.2*a*)
- Front lunge with overhead lift (see figure 10.2*b*)
- Side lunge with low reach (see figure 10.2*c*)

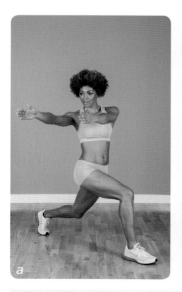 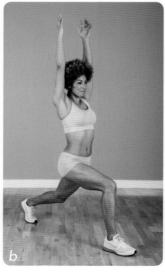 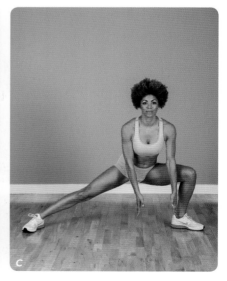

Figure 10.2   Lunges with an added component to strengthen the glutes and stretch the hip flexors.

Now let's consider specific injuries associated with common workout activities.

Cycling

If you notice pain below your knee when walking down stairs, you could be suffering from patellar tendonitis, inflammation usually caused by repeated stretching of the tendon through excessive straightening of the leg. You can find relief by strengthening the vastus medialis muscle: Practise just the last portion of the movement on a seated leg-extension machine, raising your bike seat and working at a lower resistance but with a higher cadence to maintain the intensity.

Swimming

Soreness around the shoulder can be a sign of rotator cuff impingement due to regular stress on the small tendons around the shoulder blade that help to stabilise the joint. There is little room to move in this area, so even a small degree of inflammation can lead to trapping and therefore pain. To reduce the problem, stretch the affected area by taking your arm across your chest and pulling in with the other hand. Hold the stretch for 15 to 30 seconds. In addition, try strengthening the area with the dumb waiter exercise as follows, using either a resistance band or cable machine in the gym.

DUMB WAITER

Exercise Focus
Shoulder girdle

How To
Start in either a standing or sitting position with your elbows tucked in to your sides and your shoulder blades drawn back and down. Keeping your elbows in contact with your ribs and your palms up, take your hands out to the side as far as is comfortable (see figure 10.3). You may not be able to move far at first, but with practice, you will increase the range. Once you can achieve a good range of movement, add a resistance band in your hands to further improve the strength in the rotator cuff muscles.

Keep your shoulders down and your abdominal muscles lightly pulled in.

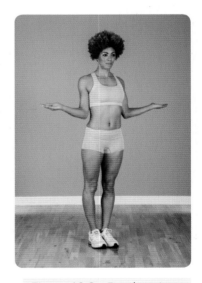

Figure 10.3   Dumb waiter.

Running

Sadly for you pavement pounders, running poses a greater risk of injury than cycling and swimming. Runners commonly present plantar fasciitis and iliotibial band (ITB) syndrome. The first condition refers to a strain on the connective tissue in the sole of the foot that is stretched on every foot strike, causing a dull ache when you are at rest. To counter this, reduce your mileage and head for the pool, where you can run with reduced impact on the foot. ITB syndrome is caused by friction between the fibrous band that attaches down the outside of the leg and the bottom end of the thigh bone. It can present itself as a sharp pain on the outside of your knee. Working the area with a foam roller is a great way to help reduce tightness in the area and so bring relief (see the cooling-down section of chapter 4 for foam rolling exercise descriptions).

In the worst-case scenario, should you find you are suffering from an acute injury (a traumatic incident) or a chronic injury (a minor irritation that builds up over time), remember the RICE regimen:

- *Rest*—No awards exist for trying to die like a hero during your workouts, so listen to your body and take a day off if you need to.
- *Ice*—Use for around 15 minutes every hour to help reduce inflammation.
- *Compression*—An elastic bandage can help to restrict swelling, preventing loss of function.
- *Elevation*—Resting the affected limb in a lifted position will assist your circulatory system as it gradually removes the excess fluid.

AT A GLANCE

- When menstruating, lower the intensity of your workout and modify your diet slightly to ensure you take in adequate supplies of iron and lower your sodium intake.
- Avoid aiming for unrealistically low levels of body fat, as this can be the catalyst for a serious threat to your health known as the female athlete triad—disordered eating, amenorrhea and osteoporosis.
- To counter the risk of osteoporosis, include whole-body resistance training sessions in your routine, as weight training increases bone density only in the area exercised.
- Pregnancy is not a red light. It's usually possible to exercise as normal for the first 3 months. Modifying your programme will allow you to continue throughout pregnancy, possibly right up to delivery. Resist the temptation to rush back after giving birth.
- Don't ignore minor niggles, as they may become major injuries. Address them with specific stretches and strengthening exercises. If you do end up in pain, remember the RICE protocol.

11

Sample Workouts and Programmes

I t's time to put all the theory and newfound training principles into practice and dive into a wide selection of workouts to find ones that meet your training and body-shape goals. If it's improved sporting performance you require, then explore our specific conditioning workouts for increasing power, speed endurance, aerobic capacity or agility. If you want to further shape and sculpt your body and generally look and feel great then feast on our interval workouts and total-body conditioning circuits for ultimate fat burning and lean-muscle development.

This chapter provides a selection of our sample workouts with tips, progressions and a workout protocol for each method. We have also set out a sample weekly programme guide to help you put it all together. But before you start, don't forget to warm up correctly with a selection of exercises from chapter 4: Warming Up and Cooling Down and then revisit after your workout for your cool-down. Enjoy!

AEROBIC WORKOUTS

Improve fitness and endurance ability with these aerobic training workouts. There are a number to try and all will bring benefits in terms of sport performance, general fitness and weight loss so try to mix and match them rather than repeating one format, which can lead to the boredom factor. In particular, experiment with different cardio modes and outdoor versus indoor environments.

CONTINUOUS TRAINING WORKOUT

This workout, as shown in table 11.1, improves your ability to remove lactic acid and to become accustomed to long distances. Use a treadmill or outdoor terrain.

This workout consists of treadmill or outdoor running and continues from start to finish with no rest. The duration is 30 to 60 minutes for a moderate pace and 60 to 90 minutes for a gentle pace.

Take care with this type of workout, as it can lead to overuse injury. The best way to follow this route is to mix different cardio modes to avoid too much of the same repetitive movement. You can easily apply this method to the bike or pool.

Table 11.1   Continuous Training Workout

Exercise	Pace	Time
Treadmill or outdoor running	Moderate or gentle	30–60 min (moderate) or 60–90 min (gentle)

FARTLEK TRAINING

This method (see table 11.2) adds variety to your workouts and challenges different energy systems and muscles fibres. Again, you can easily transfer it to the pool and bike. Use a treadmill or outdoor terrain. Cardio machines usually incorporate a fartlek option, referred to as the random programme. If yours does not, select the manual setting and then change the speed, incline or resistance at irregular intervals.

This workout consists of running outdoors or on a treadmill for 30 minutes, varying from a jog up to a sprint. During the 30 minutes, include five fast-pace runs for 60 seconds each and five sprints for 30 seconds each, at random intervals and in any order. The incline should vary in ad hoc fashion, so just go with the environment for outdoor running or change the incline after each faster period on the treadmill. To recover, run at a slower pace; again, vary the times before your next burst of speed rather than resting at set times.

Table 11.2   Fartlek Training Workout

Exercise	Duration	Pace	Time	Incline
Running	30 min	Varying from jog through to sprint	Working from a slow jog, add 5 × 60 sec fast pace and 5 × 30 sec sprinting at random intervals and in any order.	Varying in ad hoc fashion, not fixed. Just go with the environment or try changing the incline on the treadmill after each faster section.

INTERVAL TRAINING WORKOUT

This routine (see table 11.3) enables you to work out at higher intensities, as efforts are followed by a rest period. It is ideal for guaranteeing that you continue to progress your fitness, as you can simply tweak the work-to-rest ratio to either work longer or rest for a shorter duration. Use a treadmill, outdoor terrain, pool or rower. Most cardio machines include an interval feature, but if yours does not, select the manual setting and change the speed or resistance at the appropriate times.

In this routine, you'll work at a fast pace for 3 minutes, followed by a slow pace for 30 seconds for recovery. Repeat the intervals until you until you reach 45 minutes. You can run, cycle, swim or row.

Table 11.3   Interval Training Workout

Exercise	Duration	Effort time	Pace	Rest time	Pace
Running, cycling, swimming or rowing	45 min	3 min	Fast	30 sec	Slow

CROSS-TRAINING WORKOUT

This routine (see table 11.4) gets you accustomed to switching between different cardio modes, as would be the case in a triathlon. Since the different cardio exercises offer slightly different challenges, this method can lead to better balance in muscle development and better overall fitness gains. Use a rower, treadmill and cycle.

This workout consists of using a rowing machine for 10 minutes, running on a treadmill for 20 minutes and cycling on a stationary bike for 30 minutes, all at a moderate pace. This is a start-to-finish workout with no rest and as little time as possible spent moving between stations. To get the most from this format, change the order of equipment used from session to session.

Table 11.4   Cross-Training Workout

Exercise	Time	Pace
Rower	10 min	Moderate
Treadmill	20 min	Moderate
Cycle	30 min	Moderate

NEGATIVE SPLITS WORKOUT

This routine (see table 11.5) develops your ability to accommodate higher speeds at the end of the session, mimicking a race scenario. Use a treadmill or a running track.

This workout consists of 3 sets of running, in which you run 1,600 metres (1 mile) at a slow pace, 800 metres at a moderate pace and 400 metres at a fast pace. Rest for 3 to 5 minutes between each set. The 400-metre section will be tough but results will be better if you can maintain good running form. Check out chapter 5: All In Aerobics for running technique tips.

Table 11.5   Negative Splits Workout

Exercise	Distance	Pace	Sets
Running	1,600 m (1 mile)	Slow	3
	800 m	Moderate	3
	400 m	Fast	3

TURNAROUND SESSION WORKOUT

This workout (see table 11.6) improves your speed of recovery. You can adapt it to how you feel the day you work out, and you can easily transfer it to the pool and bike. You'll need a treadmill, outdoor terrain, swimming pool or a cycle.

This workout consists of running 800 metres for 5 to 8 reps. Set a timer for 5 minutes and, once you complete the distance, rest until the time is up. This means that if you run faster, you get to rest for longer. To achieve optimum gain from this format, vary the way you use it. On some workouts, focus on a fast run and a long rest; other times, opt for a slower run and a shorter rest.

Table 11.6   Turnaround Session Workout

Exercise	Time	Distance	Rest time	Reps
Running	5 min	800 m	On completing the distance, rest until the 5 min are up. If you run faster, you get to rest for longer.	5–8

ANAEROBIC WORKOUTS

The following anaerobic workouts use the interval training method with a selection of different exercise modalities. You can choose between those sessions focused on short speed work and those favouring speed endurance, depending on your sporting or fitness requirements.

BACK-TO-BACK RUNNING SPRINTS WORKOUT

This workout (see table 11.7) develops speed and fast recovery. It is suitable for athletes, games players and those wanting a short, effective fat-burning workout. Use a synthetic athletics track or an area of flat grass.

Mark out 60 metres on a running track or area of grass. Sprint from one mark to the next, slowing down only when you cross your finish line or marker. Turn around immediately and walk back to your finish marker, preparing to sprint back in the other direction after 10 to 20 seconds. Drive hard with both arms and legs to get up to speed as quickly as possible from your starting mark. Work for good range and leg speed.

Table 11.7   Back-to-Back Running Sprints Workout

Exercise	Distance	Sets	Reps	Rest interval
Running sprint	60 m	3–4	4–6	10–20 sec

INCLINE TREADMILL SPRINT WORKOUT

This workout (see table 11.8) is the ultimate hill-sprint challenge to push your limits, as well as your speed and power following short recoveries. It is suitable for sprint and games athletes and those wanting to strengthen and shape their legs and bum whilst blasting calories. Use a treadmill.

Straddle the belt of the treadmill, placing your feet on the outer edges of the machine so you are not touching the treadmill belt. Use the controls to bring the treadmill up to your starting speed and gradient. Supporting yourself with the handlebars, step onto the moving treadmill and begin your first sprint. After 30 seconds (watch the console timer and keep it running throughout), grip the handlebars again and step off the belt onto the

Table 11.8   Incline Treadmill Sprint Workout

Exercise	Time	Speed	Incline	Sets	Reps	Rest interval
Treadmill running sprint	30 sec	13–17 km/h	4%–6%	1	10–20	30 sec

outer edges of the treadmill to rest between efforts. Repeat. It is a good idea to practice stepping onto a moving treadmill before you begin your session and to learn to do this quickly without holding on to the handlebars for too long. Aim to increase the treadmill speed every 2 or 3 sprints and to increase the number of sprints you perform as you become fitter.

BIKE SPRINT EFFORT SESSION WORKOUT

This workout (see table 11.9) exercises your lower body and improves your lactate tolerance. It is suitable for track and road cyclists who need to be efficient at clearing lactic acid and for anyone who wants to develop strong, shapely, powerful legs. Use a stationary bike.

Perform a series of sprint efforts as indicated in table 11.9. Using either a rolling or stationary start, begin your first effort and get up to speed fast. Aim for 100 to 140 revolutions per minute (rpm) for each sprint, using resistance as required to maintain this rpm. On completion of each effort, reduce the bike resistance and turn your legs over slowly, or simply stop pedalling and press the pause button. If your bike is slow to restart, maintain an active recovery during this time. Repeat the series of sprints, moving continuously through your sets. Stay in the saddle for this session to isolate the use of your legs, avoiding any body rocking that can occur when you get out of the saddle.

Table 11.9   Bike Sprint Effort Session Workout

Exercise	Time	Speed	Sets	Rest interval
Bike sprint 1	60 sec	100–140 rpm	3–5	45 sec
Bike sprint 2	45 sec	100–140 rpm	3–5	30 sec
Bike sprint 3	30 sec	100–140 rpm	3–5	15 sec
Bike sprint 4	15 sec	100–140 rpm	3–5	60 sec

TRACK SPRINT PYRAMID SESSION WORKOUT

This workout (see table 11.10) is all about speed endurance training. It is suitable for track athletes who race distances between 100 and 400 metres and ladies wanting a challenging and prescriptive running session that will shape and tone their legs to perfection. Use a synthetic or grass running track or mark out distances on a field.

Sprint the designated distances, as shown in table 11.10, at close to maximum speed to complete a pyramid of efforts. Walk slowly between sprints for an active recovery. This movement helps flush the lactate from your muscles, aiding the speed of your recovery. Aim to improve and maintain your speed across the sprints whilst reducing your rest interval with every 3 or 4 sessions completed. Maintain good sprint technique during the latter part of each run and session.

Time and record each sprint so you can monitor your improvements in speed over the coming weeks. You are aiming to complete the last sprint effort in a time no less than 1 second slower than the first sprint. The longer recovery time will allow for greater lactate removal and thus better maintenance of speed, but work to maintain and improve speed and use shorter recovery times as the weeks progress.

Table 11.10 Track Sprint Pyramid Session Workout

Exercise	Distance	Speed	Sets	Rest interval
Sprint 1	200 m	80–90% max	1	3–5 min
Sprint 2	250 m	80–90% max	1	3–5 min
Sprint 3	300 m	80–90% max	1	3–5 min
Sprint 4	250 m	80–90% max	1	3–5 min
Sprint 5	200 m	80–90% max	1	3–5 min

SPINNING SESSION WORKOUT

This general fitness workout (see table 11.11) provides fun and versatility whilst generating speed and leg strength and improving lactate tolerance. It is also suitable for those new to interval training, since it allows you to attempt the intervals at your own level. Use a spin-style bike, preferably, or any stationary bike ergometer.

Start your timer and begin to cycle at a steady pace. Cycle for 20 to 30 minutes, performing periodic efforts for 10 to 60 seconds, such as sprints, seated climbs, out-of-seat climbs and hovers (elevate the bottom slightly above your seat). Perform 10 to 20 efforts during the session, incorporating a mix of different efforts described. For example, you may incorporate

Table 11.11 Spinning Session Workout

Exercise	Total time	Interval time	Interval type	Rest interval
Spinning	20–30 min	10–60 sec	Sprints Seated climbs Out-of-seat climbs Hovers	10–120 sec

5 × 20-second sprints, 5 × 30-second steady hovers and 5 × 60-second hill climbs within your workout. Ride light between efforts, adjust the resistance throughout and vary the interval times. Perform a greater number of efforts as you become fitter and stronger. Determine your effort speed, time and type as you see fit, and have fun!

STAIR CLIMB WORKOUT

This workout (see table 11.12) is perfect for developing general quickness and foot speed whilst getting a great workout. It's suitable for games players, track athletes and those wanting to work and shape a pert bottom! Use a set of 30 to 50 stairs or steps. Look out for stairs at a stadium, local outdoor stairway or a stairwell in a building.

Stand at the foot of the stairs and sprint to the top, covering one, two or three steps with each stride. Assist the movement with your arms and extend at your foot, ankle, knees and hips with every stride. Taking single-step strides develops leg speed, whilst taking double- and triple-step strides develops leg power and strength so choose which is desirable for you. On reaching the top of the stairs, immediately turn around and jog slowly to the bottom for an active recovery. Repeat for all reps.

Table 11.12   **Stair Climb Workout**

Exercise	Steps	Reps	Sets	Rest interval
Stair climb	30–50	10	1 or 2	30 sec between reps; 2 min between sets

SWIM SPRINT WORKOUT

This routine (see table 11.13) is for swimming speed work. It is suitable for swimmers who want to improve their race times, but it's also great for anyone wanting a non-weight-bearing anaerobic workout. This may be of interest if you are recovering from or managing an impact-related injury. Use a 25-metre or 50-metre swimming pool.

Swim your chosen stroke over a set interval distance at 95 percent of your maximum speed. Rest and repeat. Aim to swim the same stroke for the entire session. You may repeat the session with other strokes on an alternative day requiring a swim sprint session. Begin with the lowest number of repetitions advised and increase by 1 or 2 repetitions each time you do the session or as your fitness dictates.

Rather than compromise your speed to complete more repetitions during this workout, maintain your speed and stop further repetitions when you can no longer sustain the speed. You'll find that with regular training, you can maintain your speed for more reps rather than slipping into a submaximal training protocol and associated adaptation.

Table 11.13   **Swim Sprint Workout**

Exercise	Distance	Reps	Sets	Rest interval
Swim sprint	25–50 m	5–10	1	5–7 min

STRENGTH WORKOUTS

The following offering of strength workouts includes routines that work both the total body and specific body parts. They utilise a mix of different equipment as well as your body weight. Pick out those that suit your needs and progress as you see yourself adapt. In other words, when the workout starts to feel easy and you stop experiencing muscle soreness the following day, it's time to push a little harder!

GYM CONDITIONING WORKOUT

This workout, as shown in table 11.14, provides strength development in all the major muscle groups. It uses a fully equipped gym that features traditional body-part stations, a squat rack and a mat (for the abdominal work). Its uses a peripheral heart action circuit, which refers to how the heart alternates between pumping blood to the upper and lower body on consecutive exercises. This results in a greater calorie burn, so stick to the order of the exercises listed.

This workout is a circuit of 2 or 3 sets of 8 to 12 reps for each exercise, with 60 seconds of rest between each set. Since consecutive exercises target different muscle groups, there is no need to rest between exercises. Simply grab a few deep breaths as you move to the next station. In order to guarantee results by using the correct load, you first need to know your one-repetition maximum (1RM) lift for each exercise. After thoroughly warming up, set aside a whole session to assess and record the highest weight you can lift just once with perfect form. Do this through trial and error for all the exercises in the workout.

Table 11.14   **Gym Conditioning Workout**

Exercise	Page	Sets	Reps	Weight	Rest interval
Chest press	117	2–3	8–12	70–85% 1RM	60 sec
Leg press	115	2–3	8–12	70–85% 1RM	60 sec
Seated row	118	2–3	8–12	70–85% 1RM	60 sec
Squat	116	2–3	8–12	70–85% 1RM	60 sec
Shoulder press	119	2–3	8–12	70–85% 1RM	60 sec
Leg press	115	2–3	8–12	70–85% 1RM	60 sec
Cable curl	120	2–3	8–12	70–85% 1RM	60 sec
Squat	116	2–3	8–12	70–85% 1RM	60 sec
Triceps push-down	121	2–3	8–12	70–85% 1RM	60 sec
Leg press	115	2–3	8–12	70–85% 1RM	60 sec
Abdominal crunch	122	2–3	8–12	70–85% 1RM	60 sec
Squat	116	2–3	8–12	70–85% 1RM	60 sec

CORE CONDITIONING WORKOUT

This workout, as shown in table 11.15, improves strength in the deeper postural muscles, leading to the potential for greater force development in the arms and legs. You'll need dumbbells, a medicine ball and a kettlebell.

This workout is a circuit of the greatest number of possible reps in a specific amount of time. Perform as many of each exercise, with correct form, as you can manage in the time available, and then move to the next. Aim for 3 circuits with 2 to 3 minutes of rest between each set. On the first set, rest for 15 seconds after each exercise. On the second, rest for 30 seconds; on the third, rest for 45 seconds between each exercise.

Table 11.15 **Core Conditioning Workout**

Exercise	Page	Time	Reps	Equipment	Rest interval
Squat laterals	124	45 sec	As many as possible	Dumbbells	15 sec 30 sec 45 sec
Lunge swing	125	45 sec	As many as possible	Dumbbell	15 sec 30 sec 45 sec
Dumbbell walkout	128	45secs	As many as possible	Dumbbells	15 sec 30 sec 45 sec
Chop	133	45 sec	As many as possible	Medicine ball	15 sec 30 sec 45 sec
Lean	139	45 sec	As many as possible	Medicine ball	15 sec 30 sec 45 sec
Alternate swing	140	45 sec	As many as possible	Kettlebell	15 sec 30 sec 45 sec
Turkish stand-up	145	45 sec	As many as possible	Kettlebell	15 sec 30 sec 45 sec
Russian twist	147	45 sec	As many as possible	Kettlebell	15 sec 30 sec 45 sec
Single-leg bridge	150	45 sec	As many as possible	None	15 sec 30 sec 45 sec
Plank lift	155	45 sec	As many as possible	None	15 sec 30 sec 45 sec

UPPER BODY BLAST WORKOUT

This workout, as shown in table 11.16, tones the arms and shoulders for aesthetic purposes and also improves strength, which can be translated into better performance in a wide range of sporting pursuits. You'll need dumbbells, a medicine ball and a kettlebell. A blast workout is of short duration but high intensity, so if you're short of time, try fitting in this session during your lunch break or before work. If running is your thing, this is an ideal workout for balancing the lower body conditioning you'll be gaining in your cardio sessions.

This workout is a circuit of 1 set of 15 reps for each exercise. Rest for just 30 to 60 seconds between each exercise to achieve an intense, get-in-and-get-out style workout. As mentioned previously, this workout is of short duration but high intensity, so choose a weight heavy enough to ensure you reach fatigue at the end of each set. You have only one chance to achieve overload (the prerequisite to making improvements).

Table 11.16   Upper Body Blast Workout

Exercise	Page	Sets	Reps	Equipment	Rest interval
Fly	126	1	15	Dumbbells	30–60 sec
Arm blast	130	1	15	Dumbbells	30–60 sec
Bent-over row	127	1	15	Dumbbells	30–60 sec
Press-up	136	1	15	Medicine ball	30–60 sec
Chest press	138	1	15	Medicine ball	30–60 sec
V sit-up	135	1	15	Medicine ball	30–60 sec
Prone row	144	1	15	Kettlebell	30–60 sec
Single-shoulder press	146	1	15	Kettlebell	30–60 sec
Russian twist	147	1	15	Kettlebell	30–60 sec
Hindu press-up	149	1	15	None	30–60 sec
Triceps press	152	1	15	None	30–60 sec

BELOW-THE-BELT BLAST WORKOUT

This workout, as shown in table 11.17, is all about strengthening and sculpting the hips and thighs. Whether you want strong glutes to give you extra running and jumping power or simply to look good in your summer wardrobe, this workout will take you closer to your goals. Beyond the obvious appeal of a firm bum and shapely legs, just about every sport relies on a solid base and the ability to generate force from the large muscles in the lower body to power up a serve, spike or punch, so this is an incredibly valuable workout. You'll need dumbbells, a medicine ball and a kettlebell. As with the upper body blast, this workout is intended to be of short duration but high intensity, so use this workout if you're short of time. Even with work and family pressures, you can still get in a great workout that will move you closer to your goals.

Table 11.17   Below-the-Belt Blast Workout

Exercise	Page	Sets	Reps	Equipment	Rest interval
Lunge swing	125	1	15	Dumbbell	30–60 sec
Squat throw	132	1	15	Medicine ball	30–60 sec
Sprint pass	134	1	15	Medicine ball	30–60 sec
Lunge	137	1	15	Medicine ball	30–60 sec
Single-leg dead lift	141	1	15	Kettlebell	30–60 sec
Lunge twist	142	1	15	Kettlebell	30–60 sec
One-hand plié lift	143	1	15	Kettlebell	30–60 sec
Split lunge	151	1	15	Step	30–60 sec
Single-leg calf raise	153	1	15	Step	30–60 sec
Side lunge	154	1	15	None	30–60 sec

This workout is a circuit of 1 set of 15 reps for each exercise, with just 30 to 60 seconds of rest between each exercise, for an intense, get-in-and-get-out style workout. As mentioned previously, a blast workout is short duration but high intensity. Choose a weight heavy enough to ensure you reach fatigue at the end of each set, as you'll have only one chance to achieve overload (the prerequisite to making improvements).

POWER WORKOUTS

The following workouts each use different power training methods. If you are new to power training, you will require more rest. We also prescribe longer recovery times when working for pure power or trying the more technical exercises, such as Olympic lifts.

BODY-WEIGHT PLYOMETRIC WORKOUT

This workout, as shown in table 11.18, is a total-body conditioning workout for any athlete wanting an overall power conditioning workout and for those looking for a short, efficient fat-burning workout.

In this circuit workout, you'll perform a series of exercises in succession to complete one set before repeating the same series for further sets. Aim to land on the balls of your feet, and work as explosively as possible.

Table 11.18   Body-Weight Plyometric Workout

Exercise	Page	Sets	Reps	Rest interval
Burpees	166	3–5	10–20	30 sec
Wide-to-narrow squat jumps	167	3–5	10–20	30 sec
Mountain climbers	168	3–5	10–20	30 sec
Double-leg calf bounces	169	3–5	10–20	30 sec
Alternating split-squat jumps	170	3–5	10–20	30 sec

BOUNDING WORKOUT

This workout, as shown in table 11.19, is a lower body plyometric workout for those who have a good strength base and are already conditioned to plyometric training.

Perform each exercise in this workout over a set distance and complete all efforts (reps) for each exercise before moving on to the next one. Rest for 2 to 3 minutes between reps of the same exercise (as indicated in table 11.19) and for 5 minutes between different exercises. Remember to use your arms to assist all the exercises in this workout. Increase the distance you cover (from 30 to 50 metres) as strength and technique improve.

Table 11.19   Bounding Workout

Exercise	Page	Reps	Distance	Rest interval
Alternating bounds	172	3–5	30–50 m	2–3 min
Double-leg bunny hops	173	3–5	30–50 m	2–3 min

BOX JUMP WORKOUT

This workout, as shown in table 11.20, develops lower body, pure explosive power. It is suited to athletes required to sprint, throw or jump at any point in their training or event and those wanting strong, shapely legs. You'll need a box or step.

Perform each exercise in this workout over a set distance and complete all sets for each exercise before moving on to the next one. Rest for 2 to 3 minutes between sets of the same exercise and for 5 minutes between different exercises. Aim for short contact times with the ground and the box to encourage reactivity in your muscles, and work for increased height with each jump. To progress, you can increase your box heights. For safety, ensure that any box or step is securely fixed and the surrounding area is clear of implements.

Table 11.20   Box Jump Workout

Exercise	Page	Reps	Sets	Rest interval
Depth jump	174	10–20	3–5	2–3 min
Vertical depth jump	175	10–20	3–5	2–3 min

MEDICINE BALL POWER ENDURANCE WORKOUT

This workout, as shown in table 11.21, is a total-body power endurance workout. It is suitable for anyone wanting a short and effective workout that will blast calories.

Perform this circuit of exercises in succession before repeating further sets. Move continuously from one exercise to the next without resting. Imagine that the medicine ball is smoking hot to encourage short contact time and maximise your throwing distance. Rest between sets for 2 to 3 minutes. Select a medicine ball between 2 and 5 kilograms in weight, according to your strength, and progress as required. You can throw at a wall or a partner.

Figure 11.21   Medicine Ball Power Endurance Workout

Exercise	Page	Sets	Reps	Rest interval
Seated overhead throw	177	3–5	10–20	None
Tantrum throws	178	3–5	10–20	None
Seated side twist and throw	179	3–5	10–20	None
Reverse overhead throw	180	3–5	10–20	None
Seated vertical throw	181	3–5	10–20	None

OLYMPIC LIFT WORKOUT

This workout, as shown in table 11.22, can be for total-body pure power (PP) or power endurance (PE), depending on reps and rest times. A prerequisite to this workout is to correctly learn the technique by breaking the exercises down into their component parts. Use an Olympic bar (20 kilograms) plus weight discs or a lighter gym bar if required.

This workout involves performing several sets of one or more Olympic lifts as detailed in table 11.22. The rest time between each exercise differs for pure power and power endurance as indicated, but the recovery time between both sets is 5 minutes. You do not need to perform all the Olympic lifts in one session. You may simply perform one of the lifts and follow it with a general conditioning workout from the strength section of this chapter. Select a weight light enough to enable you to complete all lifts with good technique but heavy enough to challenge you so you would not be able to do one more lift than specified. This may require some testing and a little trial and error to begin with. Aim to increase the weight you can lift every 2 or 3 sessions. Always perform these Olympic lifts at the beginning of a training session to prevent any neural and muscular fatigue, which can compromise your technique and safety.

Table 11.22 Olympic Lift Workout

Exercise	Page	Sets	Reps	Rest interval
Power clean	182	3–5	1–3 (PP) 5–15 (PE)	1–3 min (PP) 3–5 min (PE)
Clean and jerk	184	3–5	1–3 (PP) 5–15 (PE)	1–3 min (PP) 3–5 min (PE)
Snatch	185	3–5	1–3 (PP) 5–15 (PE)	1–3 min (PP) 3–5 min (PE)

SLED SPRINT WORKOUT

This workout, as shown in table 11.23, is for short-term power production and suits athletes and games players who need to make short, fast sprints and move loads quickly. Two different types of sled exercises are offered here. Alternate your chosen sled exercise each week or perform both on different days of the same week. Don't exceed more than two sled sprint workouts per week, and allow adequate recovery between these workouts. You can use a sled with harness, weights disc with a rope attached, small car for the sled pushes or a partner as your human resistance.

These workouts involve pulling or pushing a sled a predetermined distance for a set number of efforts (reps), and then repeating additional sets. Select a sled weight or load with weight that allows you to complete the session with nothing to spare. Maintain a forward lean position throughout the exercise, avoiding bending at the hip, for maximum transfer of power.

Table 11.23 Sled Sprint Workout

Exercise	Page	Sets	Reps	Distance	Rest interval
Sled pull sprint or sled/car push sprint	188	3–5	3	30–50 m	2–3 min between reps; 5–10 min between sets.

AGILITY WORKOUTS

These workouts are fun and effective, and they are suited to games players as well as fitness enthusiasts wanting to add some variety whilst improving fitness. Perform alone or in combination with other workouts from this section and see your co-ordination, reactions and fitness soar.

LINEAR PACE CHANGE WORKOUT

This workout (see table 11.24) develops the ability to accelerate in response to an external stimulus. Use a treadmill, outdoor terrain, cycle or pool.

This workout consists of running, cycling, swimming or rowing for 30 to 60 minutes. When you pass a marker (i.e., physical markers such as trees and lampposts) or hear a cue (specific words on your MP3), sprint for 10 seconds, then return to your continuous comfortable pace. Try to respond as quickly as you can to your cue, aiming for terminal velocity in as short a time as possible. Strive for smooth acceleration and deceleration.

Table 11.24   Linear Pace Change Workout

Exercise	Time	Reps	Rest interval
Running, cycling, swimming, rowing	30–60 min	Variable	Since the fast bursts will be in response to a random cue, recovery periods will vary.

HULA HOOPING WORKOUT

This workout (see table 11.25) improves co-ordination skills and ability to move with rhythm. Use a weighted hula hoop if available.

This workout consists of hula hooping for 20 to 30 minutes using different tempos of music to work at varying speeds. Take a rest as needed, usually when you drop the hoop! Pick it up and crack on immediately. Note that using a weighted hoop will help you develop core strength.

Table 11.25   Hula Hooping Workout

Exercise	Page	Time	Pace
Hula hooping	194	20–30 min	Use different tempo music tracks to prompt you to work at varying speeds.

POWER HOPPING WORKOUT

This workout (see table 11.26) enhances dynamic balance, enabling you to control multidirectional movement, thus improving your sports performance and reducing injury risk.

It consists of power hopping for 12 reps and then switching to the other leg. Since one leg will rest while the other is working, there is no assigned rest time. Progression can be provided with a weighted vest. Don't get stuck in a routine—vary directional challenges by going around the clock or the points of a compass, returning to the centre between each point.

Table 11.26   Power Hopping Workout

Exercise	Page	Reps	Sets	Rest interval
Power hopping	194	12, then swap to the other leg for 12	5	None, as 1 leg will rest while the other is working.

LADDER DRILL WORKOUT

For this workout (see table 11.27), use a soft ladder (or homemade version). The focus differs based on the exercise being performed:

- *High knee lift*—improves foot speed and co-ordination.
- *Low knee lift*—helps increase leg speed.
- *Lateral step*—develops kinaesthetic awareness and improves strength in the knees and ankles, so helping to reduce risk of injury.
- *Lateral shuffle*—improves lateral speed transitions.
- *In–out jump*—strengthens the legs, improves balance and speeds up reactions.
- *In–out hop*—develops explosive movement in a lateral plane.
- *Ski jumps*—teach you to land efficiently, so reducing risk of impact injury to the lower limbs.

Work the length of the ladder and perform the series of exercises for 10 reps. To recover, walk back around the side of the ladder to start from the same entry point on the next rep or exercise. Use imagery to get the most from these exercises (e.g., picture a feather when you land and think of a spring being released when you take off). On the lateral step and lateral shuffle, remember to face the opposite way on alternate repetitions.

Table 11.27 **Ladder Drill Workout**

Exercise	Page	Reps	Rest interval
High knee lift	196	10	Walk around ladder
Low knee lift	196	10	Walk around ladder
Lateral step	196	10	Walk around ladder
Lateral shuffle	196	10	Walk around ladder
In–out jump	196	10	Walk around ladder
In–out hop	196	10	Walk around ladder
Ski jumps	196	10	Walk around ladder

CUTTING WORKOUT

This workout (see table 11.28) develops the ability to change direction without losing speed. Use cones or homemade markers.

Perform 10 reps of each exercise for 10 to 20 metres, resting for 30 seconds of rest between set. Be precise; don't overrun the markers and aim for smooth transitions.

Table 11.28 **Cutting Workout**

Exercise	Page	Distance	Reps	Rest interval
Linear runs	197	10–20 m	10	30 sec
Lateral runs	197	10–20 m	10	30 sec
Slalom	197	10–20 m	10	30 sec
Zigzag	197	10–20 m	10	30 sec
Square	197	10–20 m	10	30 sec

REACTION BALL WORKOUT

This workout (see table 11.29) sharpens your reflexes. Use a reaction ball or rugby ball.

Bounce a reaction ball in several different ways for 10 minutes each. This is a continuous drill, so aim to keep a high pace throughout the 10 minutes. If the ball gets loose, retrieve the ball as quickly as you can.

Table 11.29   Reaction Ball Workout

Exercise	Page	Duration	Rest between exercises
Bounce against a flat surface (e.g., a wall)	199	10 min	2 min
Bounce against an uneven surface (e.g., a tree)	199	10 min	2 min
Bounce to a partner (5–10 m apart)	199	10 min	2 min

SKIPPING WORKOUT

This workout (see table 11.30) improves co-ordination skills. You'll need a skipping rope.

This workout consists of 5 sets of several different skipping exercises. Perform each exercise for 1 minute, resting for 10 seconds in between. Try not to think too much about jumping; focus on the foot pattern, and your body will naturally begin to synchronise to a rhythm.

Table 11.30   Skipping Workout

Exercise	Page	Duration	Sets	Rest interval
Basic skip	198	1 min	5	10 sec
Crossover	198	1 min	5	10 sec
Side to side	198	1 min	5	10 sec
Twist	198	1 min	5	10 sec
Jog	199	1 min	5	10 sec
Skipping jacks	199	1 min	5	10 sec

SAMPLE PROGRAMMES

Now that you're armed with a wide selection of sample workouts, you can create a training programme to include those workouts best suited to you and schedule them on appropriate days to achieve the best results. Different training goals will require a different mix of workouts across any given week, so we've set out a programme guide for the goals of (a) improving endurance, (b) building strength and power, (c) improving games playing fitness and skills and (d) focusing on general fitness and weight loss. The sample programmes provided in tables 11.31-11.34 utilise a selection of our sample workouts.

Table 11.31   Sample Endurance Training Programme

Monday	Tuesday	Wednesday	Thursday	Friday	Saturday	Sunday
Aerobic workout: fartlek session	Strength workout: core conditioning	Aerobic workout: interval session	Rest	Aerobic workout: continuous training (moderate)	Power workout: medicine ball endurance circuit	Rest or aerobic workout: continuous training (gentle) + stretch

Table 11.32   Sample Programme for Strength and Power Training

Monday	Tuesday	Wednesday	Thursday	Friday	Saturday	Sunday
Strength workout: gym conditioning	Anaerobic workout: bike sprint effort session	Strength workout: upper body blast + core conditioning circuit	Rest	Power workout: box jump session + medicine ball power endurance session	Power workout: Olympic lifts + anaerobic training: stair climbs	Rest + stretch

Table 11.33   Sample Games Player Programme

Monday	Tuesday	Wednesday	Thursday	Friday	Saturday	Sunday
Anaerobic workout: back-to-back running sprints	Agility workout: ladder drills + skipping	Strength workout: below-the-belt blast workout	Rest	Agility workout: linear pace change	Anaerobic workout: stair climbs + agility workout: reaction ball	Rest + stretch

Table 11.34   **Sample Programme for General Fitness and Weight Loss**

Monday	Tuesday	Wednesday	Thursday	Friday	Saturday	Sunday
Aerobic workout: continuous training moderate + power workout: body-weight plyometric circuit	Strength training: upper body blast + anaerobic workout: spinning session	Strength workout: core conditioning circuit	Rest	Anaerobic workout: back-to-back running sprints	Strength workout: below-the-belt blast workout + aerobic workout: cross-training workout	Rest + stretch

Please adapt these sample programmes according to your training level and choose your preferred or required exercise modality where necessary. Remember to take at least one day each week for rest, which is essential for adaptation and progression. We hope you enjoy our workouts and experience the improvements in fitness, performance and body shape you desire.

12

Training Diary

You have probably heard the saying that the difference between ordinary and extraordinary is just that little 'extra'. Elite sportswomen often talk of comparatively tiny details that are the deciding factor between good and great performances on the track, pitch or court. In fact, you may recall the recent successful marketing campaign by a very well-known energy drink manufacturer that focused on images of events being won by just inches (or, as they went to great pains to point out, the length of one of their drink's bottles!). Since we found a lot of the information in this book from delving into the armoury of professional sportswomen to borrow principles from their training for sport, why stop at the purely physical? Competing at a decent level in any sport requires a good mental approach as well. This is mirrored in training programmes. One tool commonly used to ensure a positive mindset, particularly when training becomes tough or when blips occur, is a training diary.

Often simple by design and easy to use, a training diary is powerful enough to give you that little 'extra', whether it's measured in terms of a faster personal best, more power on your serve or fewer pounds when you stand on your bathroom scales.

BENEFITS OF A TRAINING DIARY

So, what are the purpose and benefits of keeping a training diary? Let's take a look.

Encourages Progressive Overload

As earlier chapters note, whether the fitness component is cardiorespiratory capacity, strength capability, local muscular endurance or flexibility around the joints, you can only progress through effort and fatigue. In other words, you need to overload your systems in order to bring about the adaptive responses at the cellular level that result in positive change. However, over time, these changes will help you become fitter and stronger so you can accommodate a greater training volume before fatigue hits you; therefore, you'll need to regularly raise the bar if you want to continue to improve. This training principle of progressive overload must be strictly adhered to, otherwise your journey towards your goals might stall, something elite coaches refer to as the plateau effect. Keeping a log of your workouts will enable you to establish a definite start point and to then check that you are regularly making incremental increases in your workouts to reach your goals.

Identifies Problems

At some time you may have noticed that you find a particular exercise within a workout, or maybe even the whole workout itself, a little tougher than you had previously. This could be due to the order of exercises in your routine. Perhaps working your biceps before instead of after your triceps in the gym will help you to lift a greater amount of weight or perform more repetitions. What happens if you do cardio after your resistance exercises? Can you handle a greater volume of work? The only way you can analyse variables and then tweak them to perform better in your workouts is by keeping a record of what you usually do. Often simply looking back at your past workouts can enable you to identify what you did differently in order to work at a higher level on a particular exercise or drill. With a constant log of your workouts, you will easily be able to identify whether small changes make the positive impact you hope for.

Provides a Reality Check

It's not uncommon for novices and regular exercisers alike to perceive they have achieved a greater volume of work in a particular workout than was actually the case. Maybe it's possible to confuse environmental heat with that generated by hard work. Then, of course, there's the debate of quantity versus quality. A training diary removes any uncertainty, as you can quickly review previous workouts and compare like for like, which gives you a realistic view of your performance. Nobody ever reached their goals just by thinking about them; you need to match your thoughts with actions. Writing down an accurate record will guarantee that you keep it real.

Enables Muscle Confusion

The plateau effect means that, despite regularly working out, you don't seem to be making any progress. This is because, quite simply, your body has become accustomed to your workout routine. The truth is, you need to do something different. Mixing it up a little will stimulate the body and its physiological systems to respond by improving performance. This is the basis of the muscle confusion phenomenon. If you have an historical record, it will be easy for you to look back in your diary to find a period where your workouts became stagnant and the same. From there you can note the changes you made to overcome the particular plateau. Chances are, similar shock tactics might again prove to be the remedy you need.

Keeps You On the Right Track

Let's be honest, we all lack motivation occasionally. Hopefully it's just fleeting, not leading to a significant backward slide. The important thing is to nip it in the bud and to quickly regain a positive mental attitude. Reviewing your training diary can be invaluable in this process, letting you review just how far you've come already. Clearly, then, if you were able to make this much measurable progress, there's no reason you can't continue the successful journey to a fitter, faster, stronger or slimmer you. In addition, if you keep a detailed diary, you will find past periods where your self-drive also began to wane, together with a record of what action you took to counter those negative feelings. A similar approach should help to return the fire to your belly.

Gives You a Global View

Going to the trouble of keeping a detailed log, including the many factors that may affect (or could be affected by) your workout, will help you to assess how well your exercise routine sits within your complete lifestyle. Being able to relate what you ate and when you ate it to how you felt during your workout could be highly useful when plotting future sweaty endeavours. More laterally, a record of your sleep patterns may lead you to change the time of your evening workout. Brief notes on your daytime productivity could help you to decide whether to train before or after your working day. Importantly, how does your exercise affect your mood? Understanding exercise types and timings that lead you to harbour a more positive mindset and enjoy better relationships will be a significant step on your road to a happier self. After all, exercise is supposed to lead to a better quality of life.

Lets You Rant

Your diary is the perfect avenue to vent any frustrations, anxieties and disappointments related to your exercise journey, enabling you to view them objectively and to establish solutions. However, your workout diary is only of use if you complete it religiously. Since one of its prime assets is that it helps you identify patterns that may have led to improvements in the past so you can again make use of such tactics, gaps in the chronology will render the log almost useless. A useful psychological tool is to put a cross in your diary on the days you miss a training session, as this has been shown to prompt better adherence thereafter.

TIPS FOR MAXIMISING THE BENEFITS OF A TRAINING DIARY

Now that you know the many benefits that can be derived from keeping a training diary, how can you make sure you use yours to full effect? Certainly, making a training diary is a personal endeavour, but these guidelines provide a framework that will assist you in constructing and utilising one.

- Keeping a training diary will help you make decisions about how to improve your workouts and will allow you to exercise and assess your emotions. It will also help you create an action plan to improve not just your fitness, but your whole quality of life.

- Reviewing your training diary will afford an opportunity to assess your strengths and weaknesses, ensuring you can construct a plan B to overcome the inevitable obstacles that the vagaries of life in the high-adrenaline, caffeine-fuelled 21st century throw at you.

- In addition to our proposed entries, record whatever you feel you really want to know and ensure you complete it after every workout.

- A melee of thoughts tumbling from your head onto the page of your diary might not prove too useful when searching for a solution to an issue that seems to be halting your progress towards your goal, such as, hitting a plateau in your workout performance. Try to find a quiet moment to assemble your reactions and emotions so you can write them in a considered manner.

- Although this is your training diary, you're allowed to note relationship issues. Confrontations with loved ones or your work colleagues can negatively affect your workouts, just as a particularly inspirational instructor or a little extra motivation from your training buddy can produce a positive influence.

- For most of us, our primary sensory filter is visual, so feel free to include photos within your journal (for example, a celeb whom you aspire to emulate or maybe regular shots of yourself in the mirror to chart your progress).

- To reduce your administration and make you feel more inclined to keep your training diary constantly up to date, develop your own shorthand. For example, C-S might indicate a cardio session featuring swimming as the mode, GX-Z could be a group exercise class (in this case, Zumba), and G-F might be a gym workout made up of functional resistance exercises.

DESIGNING YOUR TRAINING DIARY

From an inexpensive notebook and printed tables found in the bookshop to downloadable Excel spreadsheets, the choice is yours. The best advice we can give you is the simplest—choose the one you'll use. If you're likely to forget stuff and you need an instant information dump, clearly a pad and pen are most appropriate. Of course, you can always transfer this to an electronic format later. The example in figure 12.1 is just that, an example, so feel free to adopt and adapt as you wish. It's probably better to start with a very basic version and to then add columns that go a little deeper into the detail of your workouts and your frame of mind once you get used to the discipline of keeping a log.

In this log, you are free to note anything relevant to your session, for example, any particular fatigue or muscle soreness, exercises you particularly enjoyed or disliked, indigestion or thirst, and whether you worked out alone or with a partner. This can be your section for anything that does not fit into a specific category. Or, as another example, you may choose to focus on a specific body part and note whether you completed a whole-body workout, legs workout, upper body workout and so forth, to avoid overloading the same muscle groups on subsequent days.

Figure 12.1   Sample Training Diary

Week Number:_____

	Type of workout	Duration	Sets & reps	Intensity	Preworkout fuel	Performance	Postworkout fuel	Recovery
Mon								
Tue								
Wed								
Thur								
Fri								
Sat								
Sun								

From D. Hodgkin and C. Pearce, 2014, *Better body workouts for women*, (Champaign, IL: Human Kinetics).

Training Diary Key

Workout type: cardio, resistance, combined, indoor, outdoor, and so on

Duration: time taken, ideally segmented into warm-up, workout and cool-down

Sets and reps: record of the actual volume of work in the session

Intensity: Rate how difficult the workout felt from 1 (easy) to 10 (exhausting).

Preworkout fuel: What did you eat or drink in the preceding 2 hours?

Performance: rating from 1 (poor) to 5 (excellent) revealing if you did more or less than usual

Postworkout fuel: What did you eat or drink in the ensuing 2 hours?

Recovery: How long did muscle soreness last, how was your sleep, and so on after your exercise?

Possible additions or end goals: You may wish to add a column that tracks your progress towards your goal (e.g., weight, circumference measurements, time, distance, and so on).

AT A GLANCE

- Even the most simple training log can mean the difference between achieving your goals or not.
- Read past entries at regular intervals and use the information therein to make decisions regarding your workouts, diet and rest periods.
- Complete it daily, be totally honest, use shorthand to make it a quick job and try to record as much detail as possible.
- Use photographs of yourself or your inspirations to keep you motivated.
- Keep track of how your exercise schedule affects your work and relationships. This is a tool not just for improving your fitness but, rather, your whole quality of life.

Choosing Your Workout Clothing and Style

You already have workout clothing and shoes and possibly one or two pieces of home exercise equipment. You might even have a membership to a health club. However, a fresh approach to one or more of these elements could be something you're considering in your attempts to improve your training efforts. The following guidelines will help you to find the right clothing and workout style.

WORKOUT CLOTHING

Workout attire is not just about fashion! If you don't buy functional clothing, you and your chafed skin might regret it. The way to look at it is not that the right clothing will make you feel more comfortable, but it most certainly will prevent you from feeling uncomfortable and may even allow you to exercise more efficiently and for longer.

You're going to sweat when you work out. The ideal garment will not leave sweat sitting on your skin but will draw it away from you; this moisture management is referred to as wicking. Not only will this be of value in terms of comfort in warmer environments, but wet skin loses body heat around 20 times faster than dry skin, so this is particularly important when training in colder outdoor conditions. Look for fabrics such as DriFit or Coolmax that are designed especially for this purpose.

When temperatures are high, profuse sweating leads to considerable water loss. This reduces the amount of blood returning to the heart, which could result in cardiovascular stress as indicated by very high heart rates. When high humidity (over 60 percent) is present with high air temperature, the body's ability to dissipate internal heat produced during exercise is impaired, and continued participation in a workout during these extreme conditions could result in heat exhaustion or heatstroke. On warm days, choose light, loose clothing that will allow air to circulate around the body; this will improve the body's ability to stay cool. If it is very sunny (that is, if there's no cloud cover and particularly if you are at high altitude), wear a hat or visor and a smear of petroleum jelly across the forehead just above the eyebrows to prevent sweat from dripping into the eyes. Petroleum jelly is also useful for lubricating the top inside of the legs or under the arms to prevent chafing.

During cold weather, do not allow the core body temperature to drop too low. In more extreme temperatures, beware of frostbite and hypothermia. In extremely cold conditions with a high wind-chill factor, avoid frostbite by covering normally exposed areas of the body. Layer clothing so that, as the body becomes warm, outer layers can be removed before the underlayers become wet from perspiration. If clothing becomes wet, change it as soon as possible. Start with a thin layer of thermal fabric (one that traps warm air but releases moisture) next to the skin, followed by a warm synthetic layer such as a sweatshirt or fleece. All these layers should allow perspiration to escape, so they need to be non-absorbent and quick to dry. Wear gloves and a hat during very cold weather because a lot of heat gets lost through the hands and head.

In wet weather, you will chill very quickly unless you protect yourself from the rain. A waterproof outer layer is the answer, but try to avoid plastic garments because they do not allow perspiration to escape, which can cause you to overheat and most certainly to become very wet and vulnerable to chilling.

Socks

Always wear socks to prevent blisters and to remove perspiration. They should be seamless and should fit well; a cotton and wool mix is usually more comfortable, and a little padding will be a bonus during impact activities.

Bra

Around 75 percent of women do not wear correctly sized bras, a statistic that causes concern when you consider it's one of the most important items of fitness equipment you'll purchase. A sports bra can provide support in two ways: via compression to hold your breasts against your chest and limit motion and via encapsulation, closely surrounding and supporting the soft tissues. Movement should be minimal, even during vigorous exercise, and the ideal fabric should be a soft, wicking material.

Shoes

An important element here is to know your own feet, which will help you determine what you should look for in a shoe. If you're flat-footed, you need shoes to control motion. They should feature denser midsoles, especially around the inner edges, and firm heel braces to prevent rear foot movement. Feet with high arches are not great for shock absorption, so look for extra cushioning plus flexibility in the soles to allow weight to be transferred through the feet. If you don't exhibit either of these, then simply choose your shoes based on comfort and fit. If you're not sure, a good retailer will have a specialist to check your gait, but you could instead try our DIY option. Pour a dusting of talc on a hard floor surface, carefully step on it with slightly damp feet, then lift your feet as you step off. Your footprints will reveal either a flattened or a high arch, enabling you to determine in which category you fall.

Our recipe for fitness involves trying different activities to ensure you achieve well-rounded fitness gains, to reduce the risk of overuse injuries and to avoid the boredom factor, so gym, classes and running will all be on the menu. The ideal choice of footwear, therefore, is the aptly named cross-trainer, featuring a multi-purpose outsole to give versatility while breathable uppers lend comfort. Cross-trainers tend to be wider than running shoes, giving extra stability, but they are often heavier than running shoes too.

When shopping for training shoes, do it late in the day. As the day progresses, your feet tend to expand to about the size and width they will be when you exercise. Also, take your old shoes to the store with you so that shop staff can see how they've worn. Try various pairs and ensure you can wiggle your toes. If the trainers are too snug, the constant friction of your toenails against the shoes can be uncomfortable.

WORKOUT STYLE

There are several different types of workout styles—in your home, at a gym or club, or outdoors. Following is more detail about each.

Home Workouts

Simply having a fitness kit in your home is a valuable way to avoid the most common excuse (no time)! You'll find it hard to justify not having enough time if your rower is in the spare room. The best equipment for you will depend on your budget and your home space, but it's also worth considering whether to opt for strength training items or cardio stations depending on your goals and preferences. Following are the key decisions to be made.

Space

If you don't have a spare room to designate as your gym, then portable items and stations that fold down are a must. Ensure you can store whatever you buy under your bed, under or in a desk or in a wardrobe. If you were to select just one item, consider the rower because it's the perfect mode for improving the functional capacity of your heart and lungs whilst simultaneously toning both the upper body and lower body. Unfortunately, the best models do not fold away very easily, so you'll ideally need some dedicated space for equipment.

Cost

Never compromise on quality to save money, because it will likely prove to be a false economy when the item breaks. Also, poorly made products could increase your risk of injury. Rather than cost, think value, because some items are multi-functional and so represent more value. A fitness ball, for example, lends itself to a range of upper-body, lower-body, and abdominal exercises, allowing for gains in both strength and endurance. You can research home workout products through your search engine, watch the fitness shows on TV shopping channels and even get great items on Ebay.

Usability

Although many people have purchased equipment with the intention of getting into it, this has often resulted in items gathering dust in the garage or being used as clothes racks in spare rooms. If you really enjoy kettlebell training, then your choice is obvious: Simply buy what you know you'll use.

Gym or Club Workouts

Some clubs consist of a single workout studio, while others may offer three climate-controlled studios, fully equipped gym, pools, spa, indoor and out-door tennis courts and squash courts. You may not need a fully equipped centre if you only want to use the gym, so ask about whether the club offers a partial membership that you can upgrade later if you wish.

The club should have various types of equipment in adequate numbers. If you enjoy cardio workouts on the treadmills, bikes, steppers and rowers, make sure there are enough of them for the high volume of members at peak times. The last thing you want is to have to queue for use of equipment. A good sign is a club imposing a time limit on cardio equipment during busy periods. On the conditioning side, look for clean gym stations, and feel free to ask if these are serviced regularly, because you want to be sure they are safe to use. In addition, there should be a functional area for core and whole-body exercises with the latest pieces available, such as ViPR, Flexi-Bar, powerbags, kettlebells, Power Plate and the TRX suspension system.

If you like taking classes, make sure a good range of cutting-edge sessions are available. You should check to see that distinctions are made between beginner, intermediate and advanced levels. Does the club have a social events calendar, and is it the sort of thing you might be interested in? Whether it's themed cuisine nights or activity holidays, there might be clubs within the club that will enable you to really get the most from the investment you have made in your membership. Will you really feel a part of the club and valued by its staff? Perhaps you'll receive regular newsletters so you will not miss out on anything new. They might even send you birthday and holiday cards. All of these could make you feel more comfortable and so more willing to stick to your fitness routine at the gym.

Service

Staff should be happy, cheerful and knowledgeable. Most important, they need to be able to talk to members. A good club has staff who give customers the motivation to stick to routines and achieve their goals. When you visit a club for the first time, investigate it thoroughly by walking around on your own and asking members if they would recommend it. (The best place to get these reports is in the sauna or steam room!) On your first tour of the club, watch for out-of-order signs; a club committed to high levels of service will not allow equipment to be out of service for very long. Are the staff motivated to serve you? Member comment and feedback forms and fliers displaying employees of the month are good signs indicating the club cares about what you think.

Price

There are varying price scales and ranges of facilities and services, so shop around to suit your budget. Often you can get off-peak prices when the club is less busy. Recent UK government intervention has prevented clubs from tying you into long periods of payment, but it's worth checking details, such as whether they defer your membership if you are on long-term disability or have to work away from your city for a period. Look out for the recent market addition of budget gyms that offer little service but have the bonus of being low cost with no contractual commitment.

Hours

Club operating hours should fit in with your schedule. If you join a club close to home, make sure you can go in the early morning or evening. If it closes at 9:30 p.m. on weekday evenings, does this give you adequate time to travel from work, exercise and then shower afterwards?

Compatibility

Do you feel comfortable in the club environment? Can you picture yourself working out in the gym? Some clubs have separate gyms for women and men; is this important to you? Most people join clubs within easy reach of the home or workplace because when it's cold, dark and late, people more likely to opt out of sessions if it takes too much effort to get there. If you need parking space, is there enough? If you have children, are they welcome at the club? If so, at what times? Is there a child care facility or perhaps children's activity programmes in place?

Outdoor Workouts

Taking your workouts into your garden or the park instead of staying indoors can liven up your senses and improve your state of mind. Beyond the usual endorphin rush that is known as the 'runner's high', a workout in the great outdoors can leave you truly looking and feeling great. Here are a few things to consider to help you optimise the benefits of outdoor training:

- Ensure the surface you choose, be that grass, tarmac, paving stones or whatever, is as flat as possible, and be aware of any potential hazards such as potholes, wet patches and loose surfaces.
- If using outdoor exercise stations, often found in parks and play-grounds, check that the apparatus is safe and sturdy before subjecting it to your full body weight.

- As mentioned earlier, wrap up with layers if it's cold but, just as important, apply sunscreen to any exposed body parts if you're heading out on a sunny day.
- Always be alert, wear bright clothing, stay in well-lit areas after dark, work out with a friend, take your phone, tell someone your likely route and expected return time, and vary the days and times of your sessions.

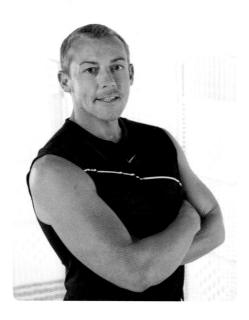

Dean Hodgkin was the resident fitness writer for *Bodyfit* magazine, contributing editor at *Zest* and a regular contributor to various other publications, including *Health & Fitness, Women's Fitness, Cosmopolitan, Weight Watchers, Company* and *She*. His writing has also been featured in the *Times, Daily Express, News of the World, FHM, Men's Health* and *GQ*.

Hodgkin is an experienced presenter, having appeared on various television and radio shows internationally and in more than 20 fitness videos and DVDs. In addition, Hodgkin regularly presents master classes and seminars at trade and consumer events in 36 countries, including the United Kingdom and United States. The recipient of the International Fitness Showcase 2012 Lifetime Achievement Award for services to the fitness industry, he was also voted Best International Fitness Presenter at the One Body One World awards in New York. He is a three-time world and two-time European champion in karate.

Hodgkin recently released *Physiology & Fitness*, a new approach to teaching fitness in the form of a combined lecture/workout DVD package for The Great Courses that provides an understanding of how the body works and so how to exercise correctly, safely and efficiently to guarantee health and fitness results. Hodgkin lives in the United Kingdom.

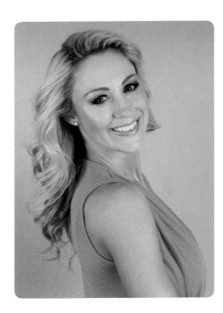

Caroline Pearce is a former international athlete and a current nutritionist, fitness consultant, model and TV presenter. She holds a first class honors degree in sports science and master's degree in nutrition and exercise physiology from Loughborough University. She has contributed to and has been featured in and on the cover of numerous fitness and health magazines, including *Bodyfit*, *Women's Health & Fitness*, *Women's Fitness*, *Zest*, *Ultra Fit*, *WorkOut Magazine* and *Muscle & Fitness*.

Pearce's athletic career started when she represented Great Britain at the age of 15 in the pentathlon and progressed to senior honors and a place in the European Cup heptathlon team at the age of 24, where she helped the team secure their place in the Super League. She is a two-time national AAA heptathlon champion and a silver medalist in the long jump. She transferred her speed and power to ice and made her debut on the Great Britain bobsleigh team at the World Bobsleigh Championships in Calgary. Her athletic success led her to become the face of the Adidas/Polar clothing line and model for sporting brands Nike, Reebok and Speedo. She is also the official spokesperson for Performance Health Systems, delivering accredited Power Plate courses to trainers, professional sports teams and healthcare officials around the world. In 2008 Pearce took a role as 'Ice' on the television show *Gladiators*, the UK franchise of the popular *American Gladiators* programme. She is now a regular TV sport and fitness presenter and has released her fitness DVD *Total Cardio Burn*. Pearce lives in the United Kingdom.

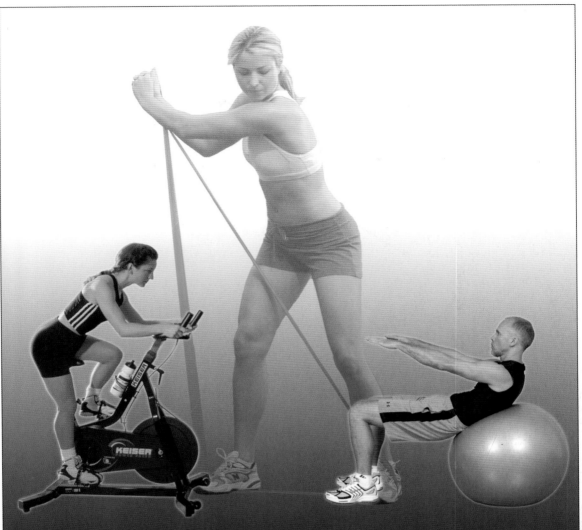

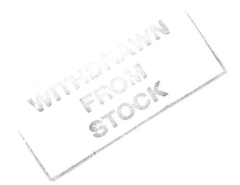